W9-DFJ-115

PREVENTION.

Natural Healing GUIDE 2002

THE NEWS YOU NEED
about Nature's Best Foods,
Herbs, and Supplements

from the Editors of ***Prevention*** Magazine

RODALE

This book is being published simultaneously by Rodale Inc. as *Prevention Food Cures*.

© 2001 by Rodale Inc.

Photography credits appear on page 212.

All rights reserved. No part of this publication may be reproduced or transmitted in any form or by any means, electronic or mechanical, including photocopying, recording, or any other information storage and retrieval system, without the written permission of the publisher.

Prevention is a registered trademark of Rodale Inc.

Printed in the United States of America
Rodale Inc. makes every effort to use acid-free ∞, recycled paper ♲

Excerpts from the *Prevention* magazine article "The Amazing Peanut Butter Diet" are reprinted with permission of the author, Colleen Pierre, R.D.

ISBN 1–57954–537–8

2   4   6   8   10   9   7   5   3   1   hardcover

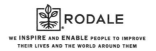

RODALE

WE INSPIRE AND ENABLE PEOPLE TO IMPROVE
THEIR LIVES AND THE WORLD AROUND THEM

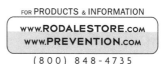

FOR PRODUCTS & INFORMATION
WWW.RODALESTORE.COM
WWW.PREVENTION.COM
(800) 848-4735

About *Prevention* Health Books

The editors of *Prevention* Health Books are dedicated to providing you with authoritative, trustworthy, and innovative advice for a healthy, active lifestyle. In all of our books, our goal is to keep you thoroughly informed about the latest breakthroughs in natural healing, medical research, alternative health, herbs, nutrition, fitness, and weight loss. We cut through the confusion of today's conflicting health reports to deliver clear, concise, and definitive health information that you can trust. And we explain in practical terms what each new breakthrough means to you, so you can take immediate, practical steps to improve your health and well-being.

Every recommendation in *Prevention* Health Books is based upon reliable sources, including interviews with qualified health authorities. In addition, we retain top-level health practitioners who serve on our board of advisors. *Prevention* Health Books are thoroughly fact-checked for accuracy, and we make every effort to verify recommendations, dosages, and cautions.

The advice in this book will help keep you well-informed about your personal choices in health care—to help you lead a happier, healthier, and longer life.

Notice

This book is intended as a reference volume only, not as a medical manual. The information given here is designed to help you make informed decisions about your health. It is not intended as a substitute for any treatment that may have been prescribed by your doctor. If you suspect that you have a medical problem, we urge you to seek competent medical help.

Beginning on page 206, you will find safe use guidelines for supplements, herbs, and essential oils recommended in this book that will help you use these remedies safely and wisely.

Mention of specific companies, organizations, or authorities in this book does not imply endorsement by the publisher, nor does mention of specific companies, organizations, or authorities imply that they endorse the book.

Internet addresses and telephone numbers given in this book were accurate at the time this book went to press.

Prevention Natural Healing Guide 2002 Staff

EDITOR: Alisa Bauman

CONTRIBUTING WRITERS: Sara Altshul; Jennifer Bright; Jesse Ziff Cool; Bridget Doherty; Adam Drewnowski; Diana Grant Dyer, R.D.; Julie Evans; Sharon Faelten; Laura Goldstein; Debra Gordon; Sarí Harrar; Janis Jibrin, R.D.; Sherry Weiss Kiser; Nanci Kulig; Holly McCord, R.D.; Mike McGrath; Susan McQuillan; Gloria McVeigh; Ellen Michaud; Linda Mooney; Colleen Pierre, R.D.; Regina Ragone, R.D.; Shelly Reese; Sarah Robertson; Douglas Schar; Martin Sullivan; Varro Tyler, Ph.D., Sc.D.; Julia VanTine; Teri Walsh; Densie Webb, R.D., Ph.D.; Dayna Winter, M.S., R.D.; Selene Yeager

INTERIOR DESIGNER: Rita Baker

COVER DESIGNER: Leanne Coppola

PHOTO EDITOR: Stephanie Kelly-Imhof

ASSISTANT RESEARCH MANAGER: Shea Zukowski

PRIMARY RESEARCH EDITOR: Anita C. Small

LEAD RESEARCHER: Sally A. Reith

PERMISSIONS COORDINATOR: Lois Guarino Hazel

SENIOR COPY EDITOR: Karen Neely

EDITORIAL PRODUCTION MANAGER: Marilyn Hauptly

LAYOUT DESIGNER: Keith Biery

PRODUCT SPECIALIST: Dan Shields

Rodale Women's Health Books Group

VICE PRESIDENT, EDITORIAL DIRECTOR: Elizabeth Crow

EDITOR-IN-CHIEF: Tammerly Booth

PRODUCT MARKETING DIRECTOR, MEMBERSHIP PROGRAMS: Guy Maake

WRITING DIRECTOR: Jack Croft

RESEARCH DIRECTOR: Ann Gossy Yermish

MANAGING EDITOR: Madeleine Adams

ART DIRECTOR: Darlene Schneck

OFFICE STAFF: Julie Kehs Minnix, Catherine E. Strouse

Contents

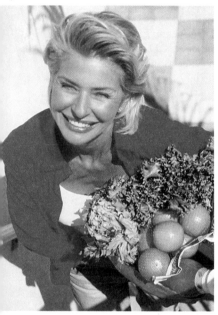

Food for Thought
Forget pills: Eating
smart may be your
best medicine.
Page 2

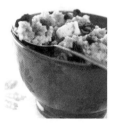

Meals That Heal
Get all the nutrients
you need, deliciously.
Page 28

PART **TWO**

Remedies from Your Refrigerator

Slash your risk of all sorts of diseases just by putting the right foods on your dinner plate.

CHAPTER **3**

You'll feel better and live longer if you adopt these seven strategies proven by scientific research.

CHAPTER **4**

Eat to beat 20 common health problems, from allergies to vision loss.

special report

Learn about the latest breakthrough in nutrition research: superfoods that can stop aging in its tracks.

PART **THREE**

For Women Only

A woman's body is different from a man's—and so are her nutritional needs. Discover the dietary strategies that can keep you feeling and looking your best.

CHAPTER **5**

These are the supplements that no woman should be without.

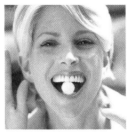

Extra Insurance
Supplements deliver the vitamins and minerals many women run low on.
Page 62

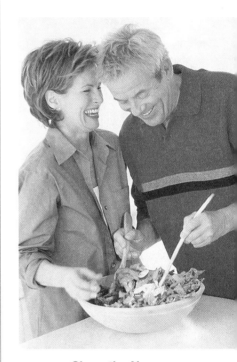

Share the News
For optimum health, the government's dietary guidelines aren't enough.
Page 34

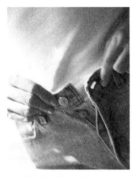

**Weighing In
on Cravings**
Scientists say
hormones may
be to blame.
Page 68

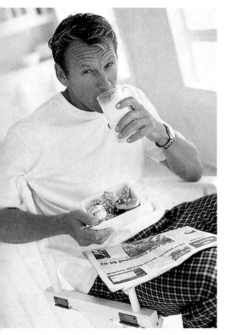

Drink to Your Heart
Soy milk and other soy
proteins can shave points
from your cholesterol.
Page 102

PART **FOUR**

For Men Only

Fight disease—and enhance your sex life—
with natural remedies just for men.

PART **FIVE**

Lose Weight, Love Life

Eat more, eat well—and still slim down with *Prevention*'s exclusive weight-loss plan.

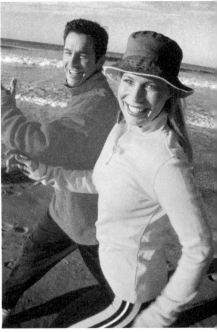

**Slim Down?
No Sweat!**
The right foods, and
the right exercise, will
melt away the weight.
Page 134

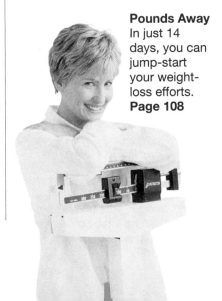

Pounds Away
In just 14
days, you can
jump-start
your weight-
loss efforts.
Page 108

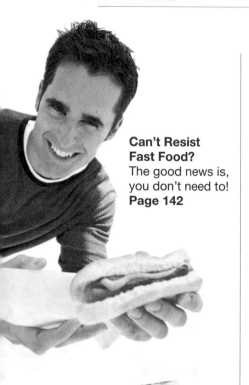

**Can't Resist
Fast Food?**
The good news is,
you don't need to!
Page 142

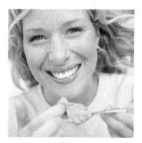

**Sweet
Reward**
Every bite
of chocolate
delivers an
antioxidant punch.
Page 154

**Peanut Butter
Lovers, Rejoice!**
Indulging in your favorite
food can help take off
unwanted pounds.
Page 160

PART **SIX**

Naughty Foods Gone Good

You'll be surprised how good these once-maligned treats are for your health and your waistline.

CHAPTER **15**

Guess what? Pizza, ice cream, and even cheese can
be good for you!

CHAPTER **16**

After years as a nutritional scourge, fat is back—
but you must eat the right kinds.

CHAPTER **17**

America's favorite condiment is good for your heart—
and your waistline.

CHAPTER **18**

Discover why you can and should eat this
decadent treat every day.

CHAPTER **19**

Add butter, sugar, and salt to your veggies—
and live longer!

special report

Osteoporosis isn't just for postmenopausal women.
Find out why *everyone* should be concerned about
this disease.

PART **SEVEN**

As Good As Medicine

Herbs and supplements can bolster your nutritional defense against disease.

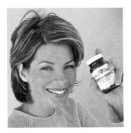

Deciphering Supplements
A label reveals a lot about a product—if you know what to look for.
Page 192

Does Your Multi Add Up?
Most contain less-than-optimum amounts of three key nutrients.
Page 196

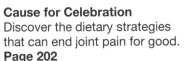

Cause for Celebration
Discover the dietary strategies that can end joint pain for good.
Page 202

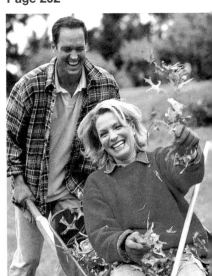

Infuse Your Life with Vitality by Discovering the Healing Power of Food

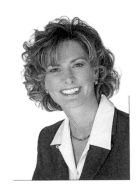

"You are what you eat" became a popular phrase many years ago, when nutrition was a still a young field. Since then, numerous discoveries have proven the phrase true many times over.

We now know that eating the right foods is one of your best defenses against disease. Making a few simple yet important changes to your diet can do everything from improve your eyesight and lift a bad mood to halt the progression of heart disease and stop the ache from arthritis.

Simply put, changing what you put in your mouth can change the words that come from your doctor's mouth. Throughout this special guide, you'll read success story after success story of real people who were able to avoid surgery, medication, and even disability just by changing their diets.

And they didn't do it by eating rabbit food. One of the most exciting recent discoveries is that even delicious foods can beat disease and solve symptoms. For example, did you know that nuts could prevent heart disease? Or that avocados could lower blood cholesterol? It gets even better. Ice cream is a bone builder. Chocolate can prevent heart attacks. And cheese may prevent breast cancer!

Best of all, nutritionists have recently discovered how you can boost your health with these sinful foods and simultaneously keep your weight in check. Eaten in the right amounts, foods such as chocolate and ice cream can even help you drop a few pounds!

And it's not difficult, especially with this guide. We worked hard to make this an easy-to-use instruction manual. We didn't just tell you the best foods, herbs, and supplements to consume, we made sure to tell you how. Whether you want to lose weight, beat chronic pain, prevent disease, or boost energy, you'll find simple tips, food plans, and recipes to help you in your quest.

We started off with a 7-day eating plan to infuse your life with the best foods on the planet. After 7 days on this food plan, we guarantee you'll experience more energy and vitality than ever before. Use this eating plan to kick off the new, healthier you. But don't stop there. Use our tips to help you solve health problems, lose weight, and rediscover the joys of eating. After all, that's really what it's all about, isn't it? Food—it's medicine. But it's also delicious. Amen for that.

Catherine M. Cassidy

Catherine M. Cassidy
Editor-in-Chief
Prevention magazine

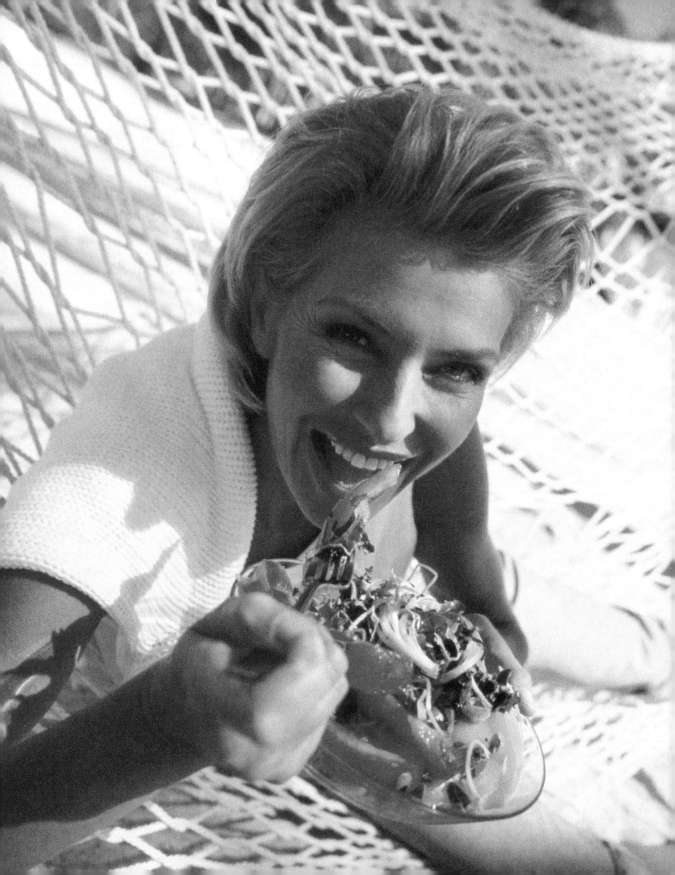

PART ONE

The Best Foods on the Planet

Variety is the key to a healthy diet. Just make sure these nutritional powerhouses appear on your plate often.

CHAPTER 1

101 Unbeatable Healing Foods

From almonds to yogurt, these nutrient-packed foods can change your health for the better.

Wish there was a pill that could help you lose weight, get smarter, see better, or beat stress? Forget the pills. Go to the grocery store. It's all there.

For example, did you know that macadamia nuts could lower your risk of heart disease? Or that blueberries could help keep your memory intact? Researchers continue to uncover delectable tidbits that hold promise for a longer, healthier life. And although the chemicals in these foods act like drugs, there's no waiting for FDA approval to try them.

Best of all, these nutrient-rich foods will fill you up fast so you'll be less likely to reach for "junk" foods that can pack on the pounds. So get started today by adding these tempting, satisfying foods to your diet. It's an easy—and delicious—way to boost your metabolism and your odds of living disease-free.

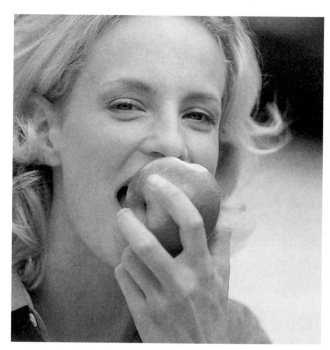

1. Almonds

Almonds are a treasure trove of protective compounds, particularly for the heart. When 18 men and women added 3½ ounces of almonds to their regular diets, their total blood cholesterol levels fell 12 percent during 4 weeks—and their "bad" LDL cholesterol levels fell 17 percent.

How much/how often: Count ¼ cup of almonds (a little over an ounce) as one of your five nut or seed servings per week.

2. Apples

Apples are a rich source of flavonoids, antioxidant compounds that fight both heart disease and cancer. Flavonoids zap free radicals, destructive molecules that initiate heart disease and cancer, as well as eye diseases and general aging. And if cancer has set in, flavonoids help stop its spread.

How much/how often: Count an apple as one of your two or more daily fruit servings.

3. Apricots

Three apricots, for a puny 50 calories, provide 55 percent of the Daily Value (DV) for vitamin A in the form of beta-carotene.

How much/how often: Count three raw or dried apricots as one of your daily fruit servings.

4. Artichokes

Even when you throw out the 60 percent of an artichoke that's tough and inedible, you still wind up with a whopping 6½ grams of fiber, plus 20 percent of the DV for vitamin C and a healthy 5 to 18 percent of most minerals. Artichokes also contain a powerful cancer fighter called silymarin and a cholesterol fighter called luteolin.

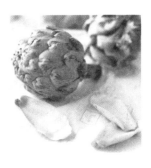

How much/how often: Count one-half to one artichoke as one of your four or more daily servings of vegetables.

5. Arugula

Arugula douses you with compounds called indoles, which deactivate cancer-causing agents. There's more: One cup of raw arugula has only 5 calories but manages to squeeze in 32 milligrams of calcium and about 10 percent of a day's worth of cancer-fighting vitamin A (in the form of beta-carotene and other antioxidant carotenoids).

How much/how often: Count 2 cups of raw arugula as one of your one or more daily servings of greens.

6. Asparagus

A series of test-tube experiments at Rutgers University in New Brunswick, New Jersey, found that compounds called saponins, which are extracted from asparagus, halted the growth of leukemia tumor cells. Saponins

Your Daily Quota

To help ensure that you get enough of the 101 most healing foods in your diet, use this chart. Meeting all of the frequency criteria will provide you with complete nutrition.

Food	Serving Size	Servings	Frequency
Vegetables	1 to 2 c raw; ½ c cooked	4 or more	Daily
Greens	2 c raw; ½ c cooked	1 or more	Daily
Cruciferous vegetables	1 c raw; ½ c cooked	1 or more	5 days a week or more
Deep yellow, orange, or red vegetables, including tomatoes	1 c raw; ½ c cooked; 6 oz vegetable juice (tomato- or carrot-based juices are best)	1 or more	Daily
Fruits	1 fruit; 1 c sliced fruit; 6 oz fruit juice	2 or more (juice no more than once a day)	Daily
Citrus/berries	¾ c berries; ½ grapefruit; 1 orange; 6 oz citrus juice	1 or more	Daily
Onions, garlic, leeks, shallots, or chives	¼ c raw; 2 Tbsp cooked; except garlic: ½ or 1 clove	1 or more	At least every other day
Beans (pinto, black, lentils) or soy foods	½ c cooked or canned beans; 1 serving of soy (2 Tbsp miso; 3 Tbsp dry-roasted soybeans or soy protein; ½ c cooked fresh soybeans, tempeh, or tofu; 1 c soy milk; ¼ c textured vegetable protein)	1 or more; vegetarians: 3–4 servings (only 1 soy) daily	3–7 days a week
Whole grain foods	½–1 c cold cereal (70–90 calories); ½ c hot cereal; 1 slice bread; ½ c pasta or cooked grains	5–10	Daily
Nuts or seeds	1 oz	1	Five times a week
Dairy	1 c fat-free or 1% milk or yogurt; 1 c calcium-fortified soy milk; 1 oz reduced-fat cheese	2–3	Daily
Fish, poultry, meat, or a vegetarian equivalent	2–3 oz fish, skinless poultry, shellfish, or lean meat (no more than 6 oz daily); ½ c tofu or cooked beans	2–3 (only 1 tofu)	Daily; 2 vegetarian days per week and fish twice a week or more
Healthful oils (olive, canola, sesame, flaxseed, rice bran)	1 tsp	5–10	Daily
Herbs and spices	1 tsp or more fresh; ¼ tsp or more dried	1 or more	Daily
Hot or homemade iced tea	1 c	1–5	Daily

not only kill cancer cells but also lower blood cholesterol.

How much/how often: Count ½ cup of cooked asparagus as one of your one or more daily servings of greens.

‖ 7. Avocados

You wouldn't think a fruit (yes, it's technically a fruit) containing 80 percent of calories from fat could lower two types of blood fats: cholesterol and triglycerides. But that's what a number of studies show—including a Mexican one in which researchers compared the effects of two diets, both deriving about half of their calories from fat.

How much/how often: If you're watching your weight, stick to half an avocado (at 162 calories per half) as one fruit serving.

‖ 8. Bananas

Many Americans consume more sodium than potassium, when it should be the other way around. But we love bananas, and they're available year-round, so we eat lots of them and get lots of potassium (467 milligrams per medium banana).

How much/how often: Count one medium banana toward your daily fruit servings.

‖ 9. Barley

This grain helps lower blood cholesterol and evens out levels of insulin and blood sugar. And good news for weight watchers: Levels of chole-cystokinin—a hormone that keeps you feeling full—were elevated for a longer period after people ate a barley meal in one study.

How much/how often: Research shows that 3 or more grams of beta-glucan (a type of fiber) per day lowers cholesterol; ⅓ cup of cooked barley provides 3 grams. Count ½ cup of cooked barley as one of your 5 to 10 daily servings of whole grains.

‖ 10. Basil

Because basil is an important spice in Thai cuisine, Thailand's National Cancer Institute included it in a study of the health benefits of common Thai foods. The study found that basil was a particularly potent stimulator of enzymes that detoxify carcinogens. Its flavor and aroma compounds, called monoterpenoids, also kill cancer tumor cells.

How much/how often: Have basil as often as you like, the more the better. One teaspoon of fresh or ¼ teaspoon of dried counts as one serving.

‖ 11. Beans

Beans can help you lower your blood cholesterol and steady your blood sugar as well as provide a quality low-fat protein source to your diet. One-half cup of beans gives you 25 percent of the DV for folate, the B vitamin that reduces the risk of birth defects and is linked to a lower risk of heart disease and certain cancers.

How much/how often:
Have ½ cup of cooked beans at least three times a week. As a vegetarian substitute, count ½ cup of cooked beans for 1 ounce of animal protein (the fish/poultry/meat group).

12. Beef and Lamb

After decades of beef-bashing, scientists are finding something nice to say about this meat. It turns out that beef—and lamb as well—actually contains a type of fat that fights cancer. It's called conjugated linoleic acid (CLA) and is in the fat of animals like cows and lambs.

How much/how often: Because beef and lamb also tend to be high in artery-clogging saturated fat, limit them to about 3 ounces three times a week or less.

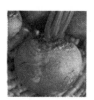

13. Beets

Like so many of the compounds that pigment deeply colored fruits and vegetables, the ones in beets are health promoters. The principal pigment is beta-cyanin, which may prevent chromosome damage, a first step on the road to cancer. Beets are also a good source of fiber (nearly 3 grams per cooked cupful) and magnesium (16 percent of the DV in the same amount).

How much/how often: One-half cup of cooked beets counts as one of your four or more daily servings of vegetables.

natural WONDER

MACADAMIAS
Research has shown that a diet high in macadamias was as effective as the American Heart Association's Step I Diet at lowering "bad" LDL cholesterol—and even better at lowering triglycerides.

14. Blackberries

If you want lots of fiber fast, eat blackberries. A mere ½ cup packs in 4 grams of fiber, more than most bran-flake cereals. Blackberries contain a mix of soluble fiber (to lower cholesterol) and insoluble fiber (to prevent constipation and ward off cancer).

How much/how often:
Count ¾ cup as one of your one or more servings of citrus/berries per day.

15. Blueberries

Blueberries are ranked among the top three fruits and vegetables in antioxidant power in a study at the Jean Mayer USDA Human Nutrition Research Center on Aging at Tufts University in Boston. An animal study showed that supplementing the diet for 8 weeks with blueberry extract improved two big age-related concerns: loss of memory and loss of coordination. Blueberries also help prevent urinary tract infections.

How much/how often: Count ¾ cup as one of your one or more servings of citrus/berries per day.

16. Brazil Nuts

Brazil nuts are a nutritional wonder. Just one nut covers 171 percent of the DV for selenium. Selenium is part of glutathione peroxidase, a powerful antioxidant enzyme in the body that destroys cancer-causing free radicals.

How much/how often: Have one Brazil nut every other day, and your selenium levels will be fully stocked.

17. Broccoli

While broccoli offers an arsenal of protective compounds, the research buzz is all about sulforaphane. Sulforaphane is an isothiocyanate, a compound that stimulates cells to produce detoxification enzymes. These enzymes zap cancer-causing chemicals before they can wreak havoc in your body. Other disease fighters in a cup of cooked broccoli include about 6 grams of fiber and about 10 percent of the DV of calcium, 8 percent of selenium, 70 percent of vitamin A (from beta-carotene), 123 percent of vitamin C, and 26 percent of folate. Broccoli is also a great source of the carotenoids lutein and zeaxanthin, which help protect against macular degeneration, a cause of blindness.

How much/how often: Count ½ cup of cooked or 1 cup of raw broccoli as one of your five or more cruciferous vegetables per week.

18. Broccoli Sprouts

You thought broccoli was healthy? Get a load of this: Researchers at Johns Hopkins University in Baltimore were stunned to find that young broccoli sprouts contain 10 to 100 times more cancer-fighting sulforaphane than broccoli.

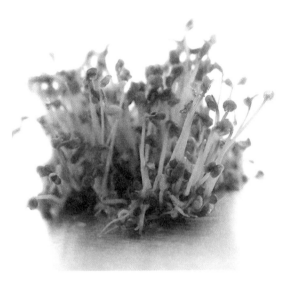

How much/how often: A serving is considered ½ cup of sprouts, which is equal in cancer-fighting ability to about 9½ cups of broccoli. Just a few tablespoons of the sprouts a few days a week should be protective.

19. Brussels Sprouts

Both human and animal studies have shown that eating brussels sprouts thwarts a major cancer-causing event: DNA damage. Like cruciferous vegetables, brussels sprouts contain cancer-fighting indoles. And they're particularly rich in indole-3-carbinol, which helps block the cancer process at its inception by boosting levels of carcinogen-busting enzymes.

How much/how often: Count ½ cup of cooked brussels sprouts toward your five-times-a-week-or-more cruciferous quota.

20. Butternut Squash

Its orange color tips you off to the presence of the antioxidant beta-carotene. One cup of squash cubes supplies a very generous 287 percent of the DV for vitamin A, mainly in the form of beta-carotene, and also throws in loads of alpha-carotene, another antioxidant.

How much/how often: Count ½ cup of cooked squash toward your one or more daily servings of deep yellow, orange, or red vegetables.

21. Cabbage

Cabbage is a crucifer, a family of vegetables linked to reduced cancer risk in dozens of studies. Cabbage is also a good source of the familiar antioxidant vitamin C. Savoy and bok choy are good sources of folate (about 20 percent of the DV in 1 cup), a B vitamin that helps reduce the risk of both heart disease and cancer.

How much/how often: Count ½ cup of cooked or 1 cup of raw cabbage toward your five or more weekly servings of cruciferous vegetables.

22. Canola Oil

While not as rich in monounsaturates as olive oil, canola oil is a good source of this healthy fat. Canola's vital statistics: 59 percent monounsaturates, 30 percent polyunsaturates, and 7 percent

natural WONDER

WINTER SQUASH Packed with beta-carotene, vitamin C, folate, and fiber, winter squash is an important anti-cancer ally. Can't find fresh? Frozen is just as nutritious.

saturated fat. And although nothing can beat olive oil's all-around healthfulness, there are times when you just don't want olive oil's distinctive taste. That's where canola oil steps in.

How much/how often: One teaspoon of canola oil counts toward your daily quota of 5 to 10 servings of healthful oils.

23. Cantaloupe

Besides being one of the best-tasting foods on earth, cantaloupe offers superhigh levels of vitamin C and beta-carotene, both linked to decreased risk of heart disease and cancer.

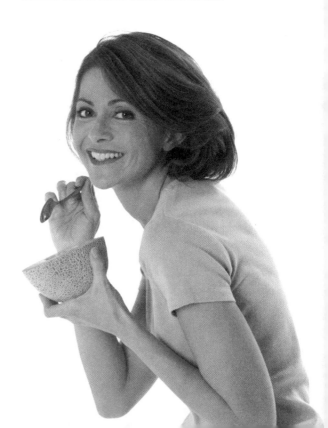

How much/how often: Count 1 cup of cantaloupe cubes toward your two or more daily servings of fruits.

‖ 24. Carrots

Carrots have become synonymous with beta-carotene, but they are also exceptionally high in another carotenoid: alpha-carotene. These carotenoids disarm destructive compounds that attack cells and alter their DNA in a cancer-promoting fashion.

How much/how often: Count one medium carrot, ½ cup of cooked, or 1 cup of raw slices as one of your one or more daily servings of deep yellow, orange, or red vegetables.

‖ 25. Cauliflower

Loaded with the standard cruciferous arsenal of nutrients, cauliflower has the potential to help prevent a variety of cancers, including those of the breast and colon.

How much/how often: Count ½ cup of cooked or 1 cup of raw cauliflower florets toward your five-times-a-week crucifer minimum.

‖ 26. Celery

The Chinese figured it out long ago; their traditional medicine used celery to treat high blood pressure—a treatment now supported by animal research and preliminary human studies.

How much/how often: Count 1 cup of sliced raw celery or ½ cup of cooked as one of your four or more daily vegetable servings.

‖ 27. Cheese

Cheese provides a great source of calcium that's easier for lactose-intolerant people to digest than milk. (An ounce of Cheddar, for instance, has 20 percent of the DV for calcium.)

How much/how often: Count 1 ounce of reduced-fat cheese (5 grams or less of fat per ounce) as one of your daily two to three dairy servings.

‖ 28. Cherries

Cherries' phytonutrient claim to fame is a cancer-fighting agent known as perillyl alcohol, which prevents—and treats—pancreatic and liver cancers in lab animals. Perillyl alcohol is currently being tested as a cancer treatment in humans.

How much/how often: Three-quarters cup of cherries covers one of your two or more daily fruit servings.

‖ 29. Cinnamon

This apple pie spice offers a surprising health benefit: It helps regulate your blood sugar. And it does so by improving the body's responsiveness (or sensitivity) to insulin. Cinnamon even battles the dreaded *Escherichia coli* bacteria, which can cause a potentially fatal form of food poisoning.

How much/how often: A half to 1 teaspoon daily.

30. Citrus Rind

More than 90 percent of the oils in orange, tangerine, and lemon rinds are made up of a potent anticancer compound called d-limonene. This compound raises levels of enzymes that destroy cancer-causing chemicals before they can do harm. In addition, a study done on rats found that adding tangerine rind to the diet lowered cholesterol. And this compound has even been used to dissolve gallstones.

How much/how often: Enjoy as much as you'd like as often as you'd like.

31. Clams and Mussels

Three ounces of cooked clams has 74 percent of the DV for iron, and the same amount of mussels has 34 percent.

How much/how often: Count 3 ounces of cooked clams or mussels as one of your two to three servings a day of the fish/poultry/meat group.

32. Cranberries and Cranberry Juice

A number of studies show that cranberry juice helps prevent urinary tract infections. It may also help prevent gum disease, according to an Israeli study. Pigments that give cranberries their beautiful red color—proanthocyanidins—may also be what's helping prevent both the urinary tract in-

fections and the dental plaque. These compounds create an environment so slippery that bacteria just can't stick, either to each other or to the walls of the urinary tract.

How much/how often: Three-quarters cup of cranberries or 6 ounces of cranberry juice counts toward your one or more daily citrus/berries servings.

33. Dry-Roasted Soybeans

Cooked and dried soybeans taste pretty awful unless they're dry-roasted. Then they can be eaten like nuts. At 152 calories and 8 grams of fat per 3-tablespoon serving size, these are not a diet food. But with all their isoflavones (a healthy soy protein) and 8 grams of fiber, dry-roasted soybeans are a much better alternative to other snacks.

How much/how often: Three tablespoons of dry-roasted soybeans has 41 milligrams of isoflavones. (You need to get 30 to 50 milligrams daily.)

34. Fish

Cold-water fish are rich in two types of omega-3 fatty acids: eicosapentaenoic acid (EPA) and docosahexaenoic acid (DHA). Both of these special fats have been shown to prevent heart disease, boost brainpower, and soothe arthritis inflammation.

How much/how often: Have fish at least twice a week. The fattier the fish—like salmon, mackerel, and sardines—the better.

35. Flaxseed

If you went looking for flaxseed a few years ago, you were lucky if your local health food store carried a packet. But as the news of flaxseed's astonishing disease-fighting potential—particularly in regard to cancer and heart disease—traveled from research labs to consumers, the food industry responded with an increasing choice of products made from the seeds: frozen waffles, breads, and cereals. Flax is also a good constipation fighter.

How much/how often: Flaxseed comes as whole or ground seeds. You can easily add the ground seeds (flaxseed meal) to recipes. A rule of thumb for muffins and fruit breads: Replace one-quarter of the flour with flaxseed meal. The meal also works as a partial fat substitute; use 3 tablespoons in place of each tablespoon of oil or shortening. Include 1 to 2½ tablespoons of flaxseed per day in your meals to get its beneficial effects. If you're taking medication or have a bowel obstruction, ask your doctor before adding flaxseed to your daily eating plan—it can affect absorption of medications.

36. Flaxseed Oil

As with flaxseeds, flaxseed oil contains healthy amounts of the heart-protective omega-3 fatty acids.

How much/how often: One teaspoon of flaxseed oil counts as one of your daily quota of 5 to 10 servings of healthful oils.

37. Garlic

Garlic has inspired hundreds of studies because it casts such a wide healing net. It protects against cancer, heart disease, bacterial infections, and maybe more. On the heart disease front, garlic battles a number of risk factors: high cholesterol, high blood pressure, and sticky blood platelets that cause blood clots.

How much/how often: Count one-half to one clove toward your one or more daily servings of the onion/garlic group. In conjunction with a diet low in saturated fat, this amount helps lower blood cholesterol and may help stave off stomach and other cancers.

Can Garlic Make You Nicer?

Next time your family gathers for spaghetti, add a side of garlic bread and see what happens. When 50 test families were served garlic bread, they enjoyed 9.6 percent more positive interactions ("You look nice." "How was school today?") at the dinner table. And they delivered 22.5 percent fewer slams, such as calling each other lazy or sloppy.

Researchers at the Smell and Taste Treatment and Research Foundation in Chicago think that the garlic smell may evoke positive childhood memories for parents, making them mellower—a mood that kids pick up on.

‖ 38. Ginger

Since antiquity, this herb has been a staple of healers from China, India, and the Middle East. A scientific review of the research named 20 different medicinal functions for ginger. The herb helps relieve pain, nausea, and constipation, and it fights infection, cancer, and heart disease.

How much/how often: Have 1 teaspoon or more of fresh or ¼ teaspoon or more of dried ginger every day, if possible, as part of your one or more daily servings of herbs and spices. For seasickness, adults and children over 6 years old should take ¼ to 1 teaspoon of powdered ginger 30 minutes before traveling and then that same amount every 4 hours during travel. If you have gallstones, check with your doctor before using ginger, since it can increase bile secretion.

‖ 39. Grains

When you commit to eating whole grains regularly, it's nice to switch around and keep things fresh. Try quinoa, a tiny round seed with a pleasant, slightly nutty taste. While it's not a true cereal grain, quinoa can be substituted for almost any grain in most recipes. One-quarter cup dry (½ to ¾ cup cooked) provides 17 to 22 percent of the DV of two heart helpers: copper and magnesium.

Bulgur is another delicious whole grain. In fact, it's a form of whole wheat that comes in three degrees of coarseness. The finest one doesn't have to be cooked; you can merely soak it and use it for tabbouleh and other salads. Medium bulgur

is good for mixing into casseroles, meat loaf, and stuffings. Coarse-textured bulgur makes an excellent substitute for rice. Like any whole wheat product, bulgur contains cancer-fighting lignans and lots of fiber (4 grams in ½ cup of cooked bulgur).

How much/how often: Count ½ cup of cooked quinoa or bulgur as one of your 5 to 10 daily whole grain servings.

‖ 40. Grapefruit and Grapefruit Juice

Grapefruit is an excellent source of potent cholesterol-lowering pectin, a type of dietary fiber. It's also one of the best sources of a cancer-fighting antioxidant called naringenin. As if that weren't enough, this fruit is a serious source of the disease-fighting antioxidant vitamin C, with 148

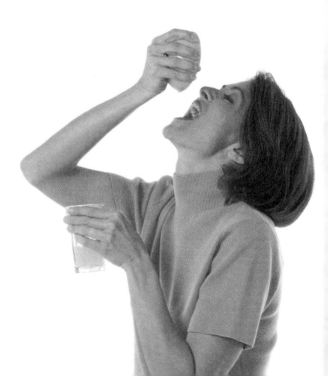

percent of the DV in 1 cup of grapefruit juice and 72 percent in half a grapefruit.

How much/how often: Have half a grapefruit (pink or red is best) or 6 ounces of grapefruit juice as one of your one or more daily servings of citrus/berries.

41. Green Beans

One cup of green beans is a very good source of fiber (4 grams) and provides 20 percent of the DV of vitamin C and 17 percent of vitamin A, mainly through beta-carotene. Green beans are also a good source of two other carotenoids—lutein and zeaxanthin—which offer protection from blindness caused by macular degeneration.

How much/how often: One-half cup of cooked green beans counts as one of your four or more daily servings of vegetables.

42. Green Soybeans (Edamame)

Next time you're in a Japanese restaurant, order edamame as an appetizer. The pods come salted, so don't eat them; just use your teeth to slip out the soybeans. You can also find edamame, fresh or frozen, in the pods or not, in some supermarkets and health food stores.

How much/how often: One-half cup of cooked, shelled fresh soybeans has 11 milligrams of isoflavones. (You need to get 30 to 50 milligrams daily.)

43. Horseradish

If you love this sharp-tasting condiment, pile it on for a dose of isothiocyanates, compounds that deactivate chemicals before they can turn into cancer triggers. That dollop of horseradish is also adding to your vitamin C supply; there's 27 percent of the DV in 4 teaspoons of fresh horseradish and 8 percent in prepared horseradish.

How much/how often: Since it's used mainly as a condiment, there is no recommended serving amount, and it doesn't count toward any of the food groups, so use it as often as you like.

44. Hot Peppers

Capsaicin, the antioxidant compound that gives jalapeños and other peppers their fire, also fights cancer and heart disease.

How much/how often: No dose has been determined, so add hot peppers to foods according to your tastes.

45. Kiwifruit

Kiwifruit has long been touted for its extravagant vitamin C levels (124 percent of the DV in just one) and its helpful dose of fiber (2.6 grams in each). A University of Texas at Galveston study found that kiwifruit is also a good source of the antioxidant eye protectors lutein and zeaxanthin, which fend off macular degeneration and cataracts.

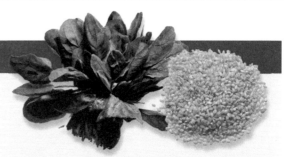

QUICK & HEALTHY
BROWN RICE WITH SPINACH AND FETA CHEESE

Jazz up plain old rice with the flavors of Greece. This main-dish casserole gets powerful antioxidants from the spinach and plenty of fiber from the brown rice.

1	teaspoon olive oil
1	large onion, finely chopped
1	cup brown rice
2½	cups water
1	box (10 ounces) frozen chopped spinach, thawed and well-drained
4	ounces reduced-fat feta cheese, finely crumbled
8	kalamata olives, pitted and finely chopped
4	eggs, lightly beaten, or 1 cup fat-free liquid egg substitute

In a large saucepan, warm the oil over medium heat. Add the onion and cook, stirring often, for 5 minutes. Stir in the rice and water. Bring to a boil. Cover, reduce the heat, and simmer for 45 minutes, or until all the water has been absorbed. Remove from the heat.

Preheat the oven to 350°F. Coat an 8" × 8" glass baking dish with cooking spray.

Stir the spinach, feta, and olives into the rice. Stir in the eggs or egg substitute. Spoon into the baking dish.

Bake for 25 to 30 minutes, or until a knife inserted in the center comes out clean. Let stand for 5 minutes before serving.

MAKES 4 SERVINGS

Per serving: 391 calories, 19 g protein, 49 g carbohydrates, 13.5 g fat, 213 mg cholesterol, 5 g dietary fiber, 677 mg sodium

---

How much/how often: One kiwifruit counts as one of your two or more daily fruit servings.

‖ 46. Leafy Greens

Dark, bitter greens like kale, chard, collards, and mustard greens are jam-packed with an extraordinary array of disease fighters. One cup (two servings) of cooked spinach provides 66 percent of the DV of folate; that amount of turnip or collard greens has about 43 percent. Dark greens are also good sources of calcium, magnesium, vitamin C, and vitamin K. Kale and bok choy in particular are high in calcium. And dandelion greens are a good source of vitamin C and offer some calcium and magnesium as well.

How much/how often: One-half cup of cooked or 2 cups of raw greens counts toward your one or more daily servings of greens. Sautéing greens in a little oil (olive or canola is healthiest) makes it easier for your body to absorb the carotenoids.

‖ 47. Lobster

A 3-ounce portion of lobster takes care of 52 percent of the DV of selenium and a smattering of other minerals. But lobster's true nutritional calling is copper: 82 percent of the DV is in 3 ounces. Indulge in an 8-ounce lobster tail, and you're getting 121 percent of this often neglected mineral.

How much/how often: Two to 3 ounces of lobster counts as one of your two to three daily servings of the fish/poultry/meat group. You can eat it as often as you like.

‖ 48. Mangoes

This delicious fruit provides 161 percent of the DV for vitamin A (through beta-carotene) and nearly 100 percent of the vitamin C requirement. These two antioxidants are champions against heart disease, cancer, and other chronic diseases.

How much/how often: Count one mango toward your two or more daily fruits.

‖ 49. Milk

In recent years, nutrition experts have increased the amount of calcium recommended to 1,000 milligrams daily for adults up to age 50 and 1,500 milligrams for those 51 and older. The major sources of calcium are dairy foods, calcium-fortified citrus juice, and certain greens, like kale. One cup of fat-free or low-fat milk has 300 milligrams of calcium.

How much/how often: You need two to three dairy servings daily. Count one glass of milk as a serving.

‖ 50. Mint

Menthol, a flavoring in mint gum, comes from mint. It fights bacteria and the inflammation of rheumatoid arthritis, asthma, and heart disease.

How much/how often: Have mint as often as you like. One teaspoon of fresh or ¼ teaspoon of dried counts as one of your one or more daily servings of herbs and spices.

‖ 51. Miso

If you've ever had the pleasure of eating a bowl of miso soup, you'd never guess that the paste used to make it is a mix of soybeans, grain, salt, and a mold culture aged for 6 months to 3 years.

How much/how often: Two tablespoons of miso—a standard serving for a bowl of soup—contains 15 milligrams of isoflavones. (You need to get 30 to 50 milligrams daily.)

‖ 52. Oat Bran

Consuming more oat bran can lower your cholesterol by 4 to 8 points, according to a review of 20 studies published in the *Journal of the American Medical Association*. Beta-glucan, a type of fiber plentiful in oat bran, seems to be the active ingredient.

How much/how often: One-half cup of raw oat bran or 1⅓ cups of cooked contains 3 grams of beta-glucan, the amount shown to lower blood cholesterol. Count 1 cup of cooked oat bran toward your daily 5 to 10 servings of whole grain foods.

‖ 53. Oatmeal

In terms of lowering blood cholesterol, oatmeal is a less potent player than oat bran, but it is still important. Whereas oat bran is nearly pure beta-glucan, oatmeal contains other types of carbohydrates and some protein.

How much/how often: Two cups of cooked oatmeal provides 3 grams of beta-glucan, the amount shown to lower blood cholesterol. Count ½ cup of cooked oatmeal as one of your 5 to 10 daily whole grain servings.

‖ 54. Olive Oil

Olive oil got its legendary nutrition status because it is the main fat used in the Mediterranean diet, the traditional diet of people in

Fiber Flunks against Cancer?

Some headlines hurt you by what they leave out. For example, if headlines have you thinking, "This fiber thing has all been hype," then it's time to separate the wheat from the chaff.

Two current studies in the prestigious *New England Journal of Medicine* made headlines, calling into question the benefits of fiber. One found that high-fiber diets did not reduce the formation of polyps in the bowel. (Polyps are tiny growths that can turn into colon cancer.) The other showed that supplements of wheat bran don't reduce polyps either. Does this make fiber worthless? Hardly.

What most news reports missed was pointed out in that same issue of the journal. Both of these studies were too short (3 to 4 years) to detect another key way that fiber might fight colon cancer: by stopping existing polyps from turning malignant.

Most important, we know that fiber fights diabetes, heart disease, high blood pressure, stroke, overweight, and constipation. And it may prevent breast cancer, too.

Definitely eat more fiber, not less. You need 25 to 35 grams of fiber a day but probably get only 11 to 13 grams. To add an easy 15 grams, try this: Have raisin bran instead of cornflakes, make your sandwich on whole wheat bread instead of white, and eat ½ cup of baked beans instead of pasta salad.

Greece, southern Italy, and certain other Mediterranean countries. These people are blessed with low rates of heart disease and cancer as well as some of the highest life expectancy rates.

How much/how often: One teaspoon of olive oil counts toward your daily quota of 5 to 10 servings of healthful oils.

55. Onions

Onions come up smelling like roses when it comes to research linking foods with disease protection. The studies are numerous, including evidence for fighting cancer, building bone, reducing asthma symptoms, and preventing heart disease.

How much/how often: Count ¼ cup of raw onion or 2 tablespoons or more of cooked at least every other day toward your one or more daily servings of the onion/garlic group.

56. Orange Juice

A cup of juice provides 161 percent of the DV for vitamin C and more than one-quarter of the DV for folate, the B vitamin that helps prevent heart disease, birth defects, and cancer. In fact, it has more of everything that's in oranges with one notable exception: fiber.

How much/how often: Count 6 ounces of orange juice as one of your one or more daily servings of citrus/berries.

57. Oranges

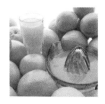

It's not just about vitamin C. Oranges are one of the richest sources of hesperidin, a compound from a class of antioxidants called flavonoids, which help fight cancer and heart disease. Another flavonoid in oranges, d-limonene, has also been shown to reduce the number and size of cancerous tumors.

How much/how often: Count an orange as one of your one or more daily servings of citrus/berries.

58. Oysters

Oysters are the world's greatest source of zinc: Three ounces of steamed Eastern oysters contains a phenomenal 645 to 1,029 percent of the DV for this mineral. Farm-raised oysters are on the lower end of this range; wild oysters, the higher end. Pacific oysters are also zinc-filled but not as dramatically so, with 188 percent of the DV in a 3-ounce serving.

How much/how often: Count 3 ounces of cooked oysters as one of your two to three daily servings of the fish/poultry/meat group.

59. Papaya

Papaya is a good source of the cancer-fighting carotenoid beta-cryptoxanthin. And papaya really hit the vitamin C jackpot: 144 percent of the DV per cup. That same amount also donates a respectable 2.5 grams of fiber.

How much/how often: One cup of cubes or half of a medium papaya counts as one of your two or more daily fruit servings.

‖ 60. Parsley

Parsley is a rich source of vitamin K; just ¼ cup covers the DV for this important vitamin. Vitamin K works alongside a protein called osteocalcin, which helps deposit calcium in bone.

How much/how often: Enjoy parsley as often as you like. One teaspoon of fresh parsley or ¼ teaspoon of dried is considered a serving.

‖ 61. Peanuts and Peanut Butter

Harvard University's ongoing study tracking 86,000 female nurses found that, over a 14-year period, women who ate more than 5 ounces of nuts a week were 35 percent less likely to get heart disease than

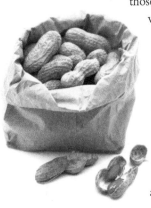

those who never ate nuts or who ate less than 1 ounce of nuts per month. Buy either natural peanut butter (that is, with nothing added, except maybe salt) or plain roasted peanuts. Besides containing cholesterol-lowering mono- and polyunsaturated fat, peanuts are rich in the amino acid arginine, which

converts to nitric oxide, a substance that lowers blood pressure and helps prevent blood clots.

How much/how often: Count 1 ounce (3 tablespoons) of peanuts or 2 tablespoons of natural peanut butter with no hydrogenated oil as one of your five nut or seed servings per week.

‖ 62. Peas

Peas look like beans but count as greens— they have much less protein and more water than beans, and they offer some of the same nutrients supplied by greens, like vitamin K and beta-carotene. At 4 grams of fiber per ½ cup, peas are an excellent source of this health promoter. Yet another nutrition highlight is worthwhile amounts of lutein and zeaxanthin, two carotenoids that help ward off macular degeneration, a cause of blindness.

How much/how often: Count ½ cup of cooked peas as one of your one or more daily servings of greens.

‖ 63. Potatoes

Potatoes are most notable for what they're *not*. They're not inherently high in fat or sodium. And potatoes can make up the bulk of your meal at a reasonable calorie expense. A 7-ounce potato with skin has 220 calories, no fat, 43 percent of the DV for vitamin C, and 4 to 35 percent of the DV for most B vitamins.

How much/how often: A medium baked potato with the skin still on counts as one of your four or more vegetable servings.

64. Prunes and Prune Juice

Prunes' famed laxative effect comes partly from the 2.5 grams of fiber in just four prunes. Six ounces of prune juice provides 2 grams, and that's amazing since most juices have no fiber. Prunes and prune juice also contain dihydrophenyl isatin, which stimulates the intestinal contractions that are necessary for regular bowel movements. Prunes also contain tartaric acid, which acts as a natural laxative.

How much/how often: Three or four prunes or 6 ounces of prune juice counts as one of your two or more daily fruit servings.

65. Pumpkin

One-half cup of canned pumpkin contains five times the DV of vitamin A (coming from both alpha- and beta-carotene). These carotenoids have been shown over and over again to be protective against cancer. As with all foods high in carotenoids, eating them with a little bit of fat greatly enhances absorption.

How much/how often: Count ½ cup of cooked pumpkin as one of your one or more daily servings of deep yellow, orange, or red vegetables.

66. Pumpkin Seeds

Just 1 ounce of pumpkin seeds fulfills 38 percent of the DV for magnesium, which is involved in more than 300 enzyme systems and is critical to contraction of muscles—including the heart muscle. Magnesium helps prevent arrhythmias (irregular heartbeat) and helps keep blood pressure down.

How much/how often: One ounce of pumpkin seeds counts as one of your 5 ounces of nuts or seeds per week.

67. Purple Grapes

Scientists are examining grapes to see whether these fruits can match the famous heart protection of red wine. So far, the researchers like what they see. In fact, purple grape juice just might steal red wine's thunder. A number of animal and test-tube experiments show that purple grape juice (white grape juice doesn't appear to work) counteracts heart disease risk factors such as blood clotting and the oxidation of LDL cholesterol, which causes arterial plaque buildup.

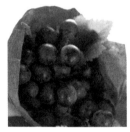

How much/how often: Count 6 ounces of purple (Concord) grape juice as one of your two or more daily fruits. (If you drink a glass of red wine with dinner, you're also covered.)

68. Purslane

Researchers have taken a shine to this plant because it's unusually high in the heart-healthy omega-3s. If you were to eat about 3 cups, you'd get about a half-gram of omega-3s. Since our diets are so low in omega-3s, every bit helps.

How much/how often: When you can get it, mix it with other salad greens. Count 2 cups toward your one or more daily servings of greens.

69. Radishes

Bite into a radish and note how quickly your mouth goes from cool to hot. Chewing sets off a chain of chemical reactions that forms the sharp-tasting cancer-fighting compounds indoles and isothiocyanates. A Polish study found that people who frequently eat radishes are 35 percent less likely to develop stomach cancer than those who rarely or never eat the vegetable. Animal research backs up the link, demonstrating that isothiocyanates greatly reduce breast cancer.

How much/how often: One-half cup of radishes counts as one of your five or more cruciferous vegetables per week.

70. Raspberries

The next time you hesitate to spend $3 to $4 for ½ pint of raspberries, think of the taste . . . then think of the fiber. In that cup's worth, you'll get 8 grams, more than in a cup of bran flakes. Raspberries also contain ellagic acid, a powerful cancer fighter.

How much/how often: Count ¾ cup of raspberries as one of your one or more daily servings of citrus/berries.

71. Rice

The traditional Asian diet—linked to protection from heart disease, diabetes, and a number of cancers—is based on rice. One cup of rice, especially brown rice, provides 3.5 grams of insoluble fiber (the type similar to wheat bran), up to 15 percent of the DV for a variety of B vitamins, and 107 percent of the DV for manganese, a mineral that plays a role in bone health and blood sugar regulation.

How much/how often: Count each ½ cup of rice that you eat as one of your 5 to 10 daily servings of whole grain foods.

72. Rice Bran Oil

A USDA/Tufts University study put rice bran oil on the nutritional map when the researchers found that consuming two-thirds of total fat in the form of the oil (as part of a 30 percent fat diet) lowered LDL cholesterol just as well as canola oil.

While rice bran oil isn't quite as rich in monounsaturated fat as olive and canola oils, it has a pretty good profile: 39 percent monounsaturated, 35 percent polyunsaturated, and 20 percent saturated fat. But researchers suspect it's more than the monounsaturates in rice bran oil that give it cholesterol-lowering power. They think it may be a compound that is unique to this oil—gamma-oryzanol—that's at work.

How much/how often: One teaspoon of rice bran oil counts as one of your daily 5 to 10 servings of healthful oils. Since it's a little higher in polyunsaturates than olive or canola oil, don't make rice bran oil your principal fat.

73. Rye Bread and Crackers

Why, despite a diet high in saturated fat, are women in Finland less prone to breast and colon cancers than other Scandinavians or Americans? It could be the whole grain rye fiber they eat, suggests John Weisburger, M.D., Ph.D., of the American Health Foundation in Valhalla, New York. Rye flour is high in dietary fiber, which, along with adequate fluid intake, pulls water into the stool, diluting the concentration of substances that are involved in the development of colon cancer and sending them out of the body more quickly.

How much/how often: Count one slice of whole grain rye bread or 70 to 90 calories' worth of whole grain rye crackers (three or four crackers, or ¾ to 1 ounce) as one of your daily 5 to 10 servings of whole grains.

74. Sage

This herb shares some flavor compounds with rosemary: carnosol and carnosic acid, both antioxidants that help prevent cancer in lab animals. These compounds raise levels of enzymes that detoxify cancer-causing substances.

How much/how often: Eat sage as often as you like. One teaspoon of fresh sage or ¼ teaspoon of

dried is considered one of your one or more daily servings of herbs and spices.

75. Salad Greens

To get superfood status, your lettuce has to be dark green, like romaine or leaf lettuce. These darker leaves have seven times the cancer-fighting carotenoids of iceberg. And more than half of those carotenoids are lutein and zeaxanthin, which protect your eyes against macular degeneration.

How much/how often: Count 2 cups of mixed greens as one of your one or more daily servings of greens. Look for mixes that include mustard greens, curly endive, red oak leaf lettuce, and other dark greens.

76. Seaweed

In a test of 68 foods, seaweed was ranked number two as a source of lignans, compounds that act as benign or weakened hormones, muting the cancer-causing effects of real hormones.

How much/how often: Count 1 cup of seaweed salad as one of your one or more daily servings of greens. It's available in Japanese restaurants (you can also make it yourself from ingredients found in health food and Asian specialty stores).

‖ 77. Sesame Oil

It takes just a teaspoon of sesame oil to give your stir-fries authentic Asian flavor. The compounds that give this oil its unique flavor—sesamin, sesamolin, and sesaminol—are also antioxidants.

How much/how often: One teaspoon counts as one of your daily 5 to 10 servings of healthful oils. Since it's a little higher in polyunsaturates than olive or canola oil, don't make sesame seed oil your principal fat.

‖ 78. Shiitake Mushrooms

Any way you slice them, shiitake mushrooms prove protective. Test-tube studies as well as studies on animals and humans show that extracts from the mushrooms fight cancer.

How much/how often: Count ½ cup of the cooked mushrooms as one of your daily four or more vegetable servings.

‖ 79. Soy

Americans have higher rates of breast cancer, prostate cancer, and heart disease than the Japanese. Is the Japanese diet making all the difference? The Japanese eat more fish, less fat, and something most Americans don't: soy foods. These include miso, dry-roasted or green soybeans, soy milk, soy protein, tempeh, textured vegetable protein, and tofu. Compounds abundant in soy—isoflavones—impart some, if not all, of the health benefits, including reduced risk for heart disease and cancer, as well as stronger bones and fewer menopausal symptoms for women.

How much/how often: No soy or isoflavone recommendation has been established; however, experts recommend consuming 30 to 50 milligrams of isoflavones from soy foods daily (which is about one serving of soy). Check package labels of the various soy products for their isoflavone concentration. Be aware that there are no isoflavones in soybean oil and barely any in soy sauce.

‖ 80. Soy Milk

Amazingly, this creamy-tasting liquid is made from cooked and ground soybeans. The calcium-fortified versions make a wonderful milk substitute, especially for the lactose-intolerant. And you get from 4 to 20 percent of the DV of other minerals, plus a sprinkling of B vitamins.

How much/how often: One cup of soy milk has 24 to 30 milligrams of isoflavones. (You need to get 30 to 50 milligrams daily.)

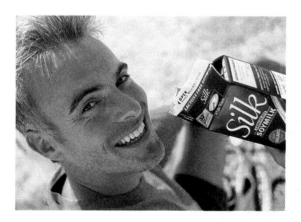

81. Soy Protein (Soy Protein Isolate)

This powder is the protein-only component of soy. Add it to shakes, soups, muffins, and other recipes.

How much/how often: One ounce (3 tablespoons) of soy protein has about 28 milligrams of isoflavones (products vary, so check nutrition labels). You need to get 30 to 50 milligrams daily.

82. Strawberries

Just 1 cup of strawberries covers 136 percent of the DV for vitamin C and contributes 3 grams of fiber. Strawberries are also one of the richest sources of ellagic acid, a hot commodity in research labs that is proving to be a potent anticancer agent. Ellagic acid destroys the enzymes that turn chemicals into carcinogens, and it stimulates the production of enzymes that destroy carcinogens. One of the pigments that gives strawberries their color—anthocyanin—is a powerful antioxidant.

How much/how often: Count ¾ cup of strawberries toward your one or more daily servings of citrus/berries.

83. Sunflower Seeds

They may be little, but sunflower seeds are a mighty source of fiber, minerals, B vitamins, and hard-to-get vitamin E. Sunflower seeds are particularly rich in folate, giving you 19 percent of

the DV in a ¼-cup handful. Sunflower seeds are also high in phytosterols, compounds that help keep cholesterol down.

How much/how often: Count 1 ounce toward your 5 ounces of nuts or seeds per week.

84. Sweet Peppers

Green, red, and yellow bell peppers are fantastic sources of vitamin C, covering two to three times the DV in one pepper. Red peppers offer an antioxidant bonus over the others with both higher C levels and more beta-carotene per pepper, covering over 100 percent of the DV for vitamin A. (The body converts beta-carotene to A as needed.) Also, red peppers are loaded with another antioxidant carotenoid, beta-cryptoxanthin.

How much/how often: Count 1 cup of sliced red, orange, or yellow pepper toward your one or more daily servings of deep yellow, orange, or red vegetables. Count 1 cup of green pepper slices toward your one or more daily servings of greens.

85. Sweet Potatoes

Sweet potatoes are stuffed with beta-carotene. What's more, a Japanese study showed that sweet potatoes, especially the darker red-purple varieties, contain another class of antioxidant compounds: anthocyanins. They work similarly to beta-carotene to disable cancer-causing substances and prevent heart disease. One cup of mashed sweet potatoes has 82 percent of the DV for vitamin C and 6 grams of fiber, plus a healthy sprinkling of minerals and B vitamins.

How much/how often: Count ½ cup of mashed sweet potatoes or one medium (5 inches long, 2 inches in diameter) baked sweet potato toward your one or more daily servings of deep yellow, orange, or red vegetables.

‖ **86. Tahini**

Tahini, sesame seed paste, is a nutritionally impressive food: Just 1 tablespoon has 1.4 grams of fiber and provides 12 percent of the DV for copper and thiamin (a B vitamin that helps convert food into energy), plus a sprinkling of other minerals and B vitamins (11 percent of the DV for manganese and phosphorus; 4 percent of the DV for riboflavin, niacin, and folate). It also sports antioxidants unique to sesame called sesaminol, sesamonlinol, and pinoresinol—all of which fight heart disease and cancer.

How much/how often: Count 2 tablespoons of tahini as one of your five weekly servings of nuts or seeds.

‖ **87. Tangerines**

Tangerines are usually lumped in with oranges as far as nutrition goes. But they have a unique phytonutrient claim to fame: tangeretin. Test-tube studies show that this compound helps prevent breast cancer. Tangerines are also exceptionally rich in another protective compound, beta-cryptoxanthin. It's an antioxidant that the body converts to vitamin A.

How much/how often: Count one large or two small tangerines or ¾ cup of tangerine juice toward your one or more daily servings of citrus/berries.

‖ **88. Tea**

Dozens of studies link tea to decreased risk for disease. In fact, in some parts of the world, people drink 10 cups of tea a day, and it seems to only improve their health.

How much/how often: Have 1 to 5 cups of tea daily.

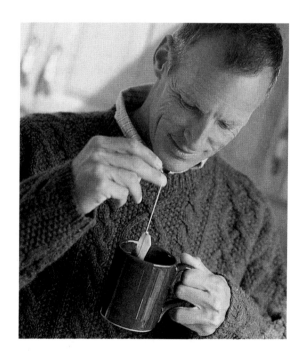

89. Tempeh

This ancient Indonesian food is a combination of soy and grains incubated with an edible mold. Although an acquired taste, it has many fans. Use it in sandwiches and spreads.

How much/how often: One-half cup of tempeh has 36 milligrams of isoflavones. (You need to get 30 to 50 milligrams of these compounds daily.)

90. Textured Vegetable Protein (TVP)

Available in granular form or chunks, TVP is a great substitute for ground beef in dishes like chili, sloppy joes, and tacos. It's made from defatted soy flour that has been compressed to the point that it changes form. Before cooking, rehydrate it by mixing 1 cup of TVP with a scant cup of boiling water.

How much/how often: One-quarter cup of dry coarse TVP has 47 milligrams of isoflavones. (You need to get 30 to 50 milligrams daily.)

91. Tofu

This familiar Asian staple is made by curdling hot soy milk with a coagulant. Tofu's blandness is its strength, because it blends well with both sweet and savory foods.

How much/how often: One-half cup of tofu has 24 to 27 milligrams of isoflavones. (You need to get 30 to 50 milligrams daily.)

92. Tomatoes

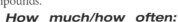

File this in the too-good-to-be-true drawer: Pizza and ketchup can actually help ward off heart disease and cancer. The credit goes to tomatoes, which contain an array of disease-fighting compounds.

How much/how often: Count one tomato, 1 cup of sliced tomatoes or cherry tomatoes, or ½ cup of tomato sauce toward your one or more daily servings of deep yellow, orange, or red vegetables.

93. Turmeric

The pigment that gives this curry spice its yellow color—curcumin—is a potent disease fighter. It reverses liver damage caused by toxins, lowers the levels of cancer-causing compounds in smokers, and raises levels of enzymes that destroy carcinogens. It helps prevent skin, colon, and stomach cancers in mice. And it is anti-inflammatory, which means that it helps reduce the risk of heart disease, asthma, and other diseases.

How much/how often: Use as much turmeric as often as you like as one of your one or more daily servings of herbs and spices.

94. Turnips

Turnips, which are cruciferous vegetables, get their pungency partly from cancer-fighting compounds called isothiocyanates. These compounds help disable cancer-causing substances before they trigger the disease. Turnips also have a sprinkling of vitamin C and 3 grams of fiber per cup.

How much/how often: Consider ½ cup of cooked turnips as one of your five or more crucifers per week.

95. Vegetable Juice

Three-quarters cup of tomato-based vegetable juice (like V8) has more than twice as much of the powerful antioxidant lycopene as a cup of chopped fresh tomatoes. Add 77 percent of the DV of vitamin C and an array of carotenoids donated by the other vegetables in the juice, and you're drinking liquid nutrition.

How much/how often: Three-quarters cup of vegetable juice equals one serving. Because juice doesn't contain a lot of fiber, have it only once a day.

96. Walnuts

Among nuts, walnuts are uniquely rich in a type of omega-3 fatty acid called alpha-linolenic acid, which has been shown to lower heart disease risk. Another compound in walnuts—ellagic acid—also fights heart disease by reducing the formation of

natural
WONDER

WHEATBERRIES
Naturally nutty, wheatberries (whole wheat kernels) are packed with wheat fiber, which is shown to lower estrogen in women. (Low estrogen levels may reduce breast cancer risk.)

artery-clogging plaque. And ellagic acid can help prevent cancer.

How much/how often: Count 1 ounce (14 halves) as one of your 5 ounces of nuts or seeds per week.

97. Watercress

Researchers gave 11 smokers 2 ounces of watercress three times a day for 3 days and tested their urine for up to 2 weeks. On the watercress-enriched diet, the smokers excreted 34 percent more of a breakdown product of the tobacco carcinogen, which meant that the watercress was actually disabling the carcinogen. Research using laboratory animals shows that the active ingredient in watercress, PEITC, is also protective against breast cancer.

How much/how often: Count 2 cups of chopped watercress as one of your five or more cruciferous vegetables per week or toward your one or more daily servings of greens.

98. Wheat Bran Cereal

Bran cereal, especially those highest in fiber (such as All-Bran and Fiber One), is one of the most concentrated sources of insoluble fiber. Wheat bran is rich in lignans, which help fend off hormone-dependent cancers such as breast cancer. Cereals made from wheat bran are naturally loaded with health-promoting minerals like magnesium (which protects the heart).

How much/how often: Check labels for the cup measure of cold or hot wheat bran cereal that is 70 to 90 calories' worth. That counts as one of your 5 to 10 daily whole grain servings.

‖ 99. Wheat Germ

The germ of a grain is its nutrient warehouse, which is why wheat germ is such a concentrated source of so many vitamins and minerals. One-quarter cup mixed into your daily bowl of cereal or incorporated into recipes provides 8 to 32 percent of the DV of most vitamins and minerals. Wheat germ boasts particularly high levels of these health-promoting heavyweights: vitamin E (shown to reduce incidence of heart attacks), zinc (linked to decreased cancer risk and better wound healing), and folate (prevents birth defects and linked to lower risk of colon cancer and heart disease).

How much/how often: Count ¼ cup of wheat germ as one of your 5 to 10 servings of whole grain foods.

‖ 100. Whole Wheat Foods

Every time you eat white bread or white pasta, you're missing out on a great nutrition opportu-nity. You get three times more fiber in a slice of whole wheat bread than from a slice of white. Same with pasta.

Don't stop with bread and pasta, however. Try whole wheat waffles, pancakes, couscous, and crackers. Since whole wheat products retain the bran part of the wheat, you get, in smaller doses, all of the disease-fighting compounds of wheat. And because whole wheat foods make you feel fuller on fewer calories, you'll even lose some weight.

How much/how often: One slice of bread, ½ to 1 cup of cold cereal (equal to 70 to 90 calories), ½ cup of hot cereal, ½ cup of cooked pasta, or ½ cup of cooked grains counts as one of your recommended 5 to 10 daily servings of whole grain foods.

‖ 101. Yogurt

Yogurt is milk that's been coagulated by certain bacteria, usually *Lactobacillus bulgaricus* and *Strep-tococcus thermophilus*. It's these guys that help us out in many ways. The active live cultures in yogurt survive harsh stomach acids and wind up in the gut, where they have many benefits, including re-duced lactose intolerance, diarrhea, and vaginal infections. It also boosts immunity.

How much/how often: One cup of plain low-fat or fat-free yogurt covers one of your daily two to three dairy servings.

CHAPTER 2

Supercharge Your Diet in 7 Days

Follow this meal plan, and you'll be eating healthier in no time.

If you want to eat well but you find that you don't always have the time to plan meals more than a day in advance, we hear you. That's why we've pulled together a 7-day menu, based on the 101 healing foods described in chapter 1. Follow this menu, and you're guaranteed to satisfy your daily quota of fiber, vitamins, minerals, antioxidants, and phytonutrients.

Each day, you'll get three meals, plus a snack or two and even a dessert. The following menus are appropriate for sedentary women who get little physical exercise on the job, at home, or in their leisure activities. If you're a more active woman and you want to increase your calorie intake to make up for what you burn exercising, or if you're a man, just add another serving of grains, vegetables, fruits, or even a low-fat dessert.

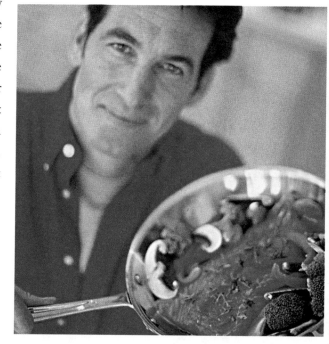

DAY **1**

BREAKFAST

1 cup oatmeal

½ pink grapefruit

1 cup fat-free milk (or 1% milk or calcium-fortified soy milk)

SNACK

6 ounces vegetable or carrot juice

LUNCH

1 cup Broccoli and Orange Salad (page 67)

2 pieces toasted whole grain bread of your choice, drizzled with 2 teaspoons olive oil and sprinkled with chopped fresh or dried rosemary

SNACK

1 apple

1 ounce reduced-fat cheese of your choice

2 rye crisp bread crackers

DINNER

5 ounces cooked flounder

1 cup brown rice (or choose another grain such as quinoa or bulgur)

1 cup Swiss chard sautéed with 2 teaspoons olive oil

DESSERT

1 cup sliced fruit (try a tropical fruit like papaya, mango, or pineapple)

DAY **2**

BREAKFAST

1½ cups low-fat milkshake with fruit and yogurt

1 piece whole grain bread with 2 teaspoons all-fruit jam preserves

SNACK

¾ cup strawberries or other berries

1 ounce sunflower seeds (dry-roasted, unsalted are best)

1 cup fat-free milk (or 1% milk or calcium-fortified soy milk)

LUNCH

3½ ounces tuna salad (the amount from half a can) made with reduced-fat mayo and served over 2 cups fresh spinach and 1 cup cherry tomatoes

1 small whole grain roll

SNACK

1 cup sliced raw vegetables (try red and yellow peppers, carrots, broccoli, and summer squash), dipped in ¼ cup fat-free plain yogurt mixed with 1 tablespoon chopped fresh or 1 teaspoon dried herbs, such as cilantro, dill, basil, or any other favorite herb

DINNER

1½ cups cooked pasta (preferably whole wheat) tossed with 2 tablespoons pesto

1 grilled or broiled 3-ounce chicken breast, skin removed (To prepare chicken: Mix 1 tablespoon olive oil, 1 tablespoon lemon juice, and 1 tablespoon fresh basil and use half of this mixture to brush meat before cooking.) Serve separately or slice over pasta with pesto.

1 cup roasted vegetables (You can buy these already prepared or make them easily on your own. Try zucchini and yellow squash sliced lengthwise and brushed with the olive oil mixture from above. Roast them at 400°F for about 15 minutes.)

DESSERT

1 cup frozen purple grapes

DAY 3

BREAKFAST

¾ cup mixed berries (blueberries, strawberries, or raspberries), topped with 1 cup fat-free plain yogurt, 1 ounce chopped nuts, and 1 cup low-fat granola

SNACK

1 ounce reduced-fat Cheddar cheese

¾ cup raw baby or sliced carrots

2 large whole grain crackers

6 ounces unsweetened apple juice

LUNCH

3 ounces baked tofu with lettuce, tomato, and mustard on whole grain bread (You can buy premade baked tofu in health food stores or the health food section of some supermarkets. Otherwise, you can just broil firm tofu in an oven or toaster oven.)

1 cup cauliflower salad: Toss bite-size cauliflower florets with canola oil, lemon juice, vinegar, curry powder, salt, pepper, chopped tomatoes, and chopped watercress.

SNACK

½ mango, 2 to 3 fresh apricots, or 4 to 6 dried apricot halves

DINNER

1 cup vegetarian chili made with chopped onions, bell peppers, carrots, garlic, chili powder, cumin, kidney beans, cannellini beans, and a touch of olive oil

2 cups mixed salad greens (try premixed) tossed with 1 tablespoon oil-based salad dressing

½ to 1 cup steamed vegetables

1 whole grain dinner roll

DESSERT

1 cookie

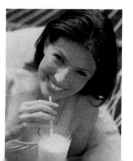

DAY 4

BREAKFAST

2 all-bran muffins

1 cup fat-free milk (or 1% milk or calcium-fortified soy milk)

½ pink grapefruit

SNACK

½ cup 1% cottage cheese

1 cup halved cherry tomatoes with 1 tablespoon chopped fresh herbs (try dill, cilantro, or basil)

LUNCH

1 cup brown rice or other grain such as millet or whole wheat couscous

1 cup red and yellow peppers and 1 cup steamed asparagus tossed with 1 tablespoon oil-based salad dressing

SNACK

1 cup protein shake made with yogurt, berries, and soy protein

2 tablespoons nut butter of your choice (peanut, cashew, or almond butter) spread on 1 slice whole grain bread or 3 crackers

DINNER

1 veggie burger

¼ pound skillet potatoes: Sauté quartered red new potatoes with olive oil, chopped garlic, dried rosemary, and chicken broth.

1 cup steamed greens (such as spinach, kale, or Swiss chard) tossed with 2 teaspoons olive oil

DESSERT

1 apple or other fruit

DAY 5

BREAKFAST

About 1 cup whole grain bran cereal (equal to 70 to 90 calories) served with 1 cup fat-free milk (or 1% milk or calcium-fortified soy milk), ½ sliced banana, and ½ cup blueberries

SNACK

1½ cups fruit slushie made by blending 4 crushed ice cubes, 6 frozen strawberries, 2 cups frozen seedless watermelon cubes, ¾ cup orange juice, and 1 tablespoon lime juice

LUNCH

1 "slice" homemade pizza: Top a whole wheat pita with tomato sauce, thawed frozen spinach, and ricotta, provolone, and reduced-fat mozzarella cheeses. Bake at 400°F for 10 to 12 minutes.

2 cups mixed salad greens (try premixed) with 1 sliced tomato tossed with 1 tablespoon oil-based salad dressing

SNACK

3 tablespoons dry-roasted soybeans

6 ounces vegetable or carrot juice

DINNER

4 ounces broiled portobello mushrooms

1 cup brown rice

1 cup bean and barley soup

DESSERT

1 low-fat brownie

DAY 6

BREAKFAST

3 whole wheat pancakes (4-inch) with strawberry topping

1 cup fat-free milk (or 1% milk or calcium-fortified soy milk)

SNACK

⅓ cup cranberry raisins

LUNCH

2 cups mixed salad greens (try premixed), 1 sliced tomato, 2 to 3 ounces sliced turkey breast (without skin), and 1 ounce grated reduced-fat Cheddar cheese tossed with 1 tablespoon olive oil and the juice of half a

lemon, with 1 tablespoon chopped fresh herbs such as basil, cilantro, or mint

1 whole wheat pita bread or 1 whole wheat dinner roll

SNACK

¼ cup hummus dip with cauliflower

DINNER

4 to 5 ounces baked halibut, marinated in 2 teaspoons olive oil and juice of ½ lemon

5 ounces (half a box) cooked brussels sprouts

1 large baked sweet potato

DESSERT

1 baked apple with ½ cup diced fruit as topping

DAY 7

BREAKFAST

3 whole wheat pancakes (4-inch) or waffles with ½ cup fruit topping (made with cubed cantaloupe, raspberries, sliced almonds, honey, and orange juice) and ½ cup fat-free plain yogurt

6 ounces orange or tangerine juice

SNACK

1 cup baby or sliced carrots

LUNCH

1 cup salad made with sliced avocado, sectioned grapefruit, sliced papaya, and sliced scallions, dressed with a touch of olive oil, lime juice, and cilantro and served on top of mixed baby greens

1 small whole wheat or oat bran bagel with 2 tablespoon reduced-fat cream cheese

DINNER

5 ounces grilled lamb chops (fat removed)

1 serving Kale-Potato-Tomato Bake (page 85)

1 whole grain dinner roll

DESSERT

½ cup pudding

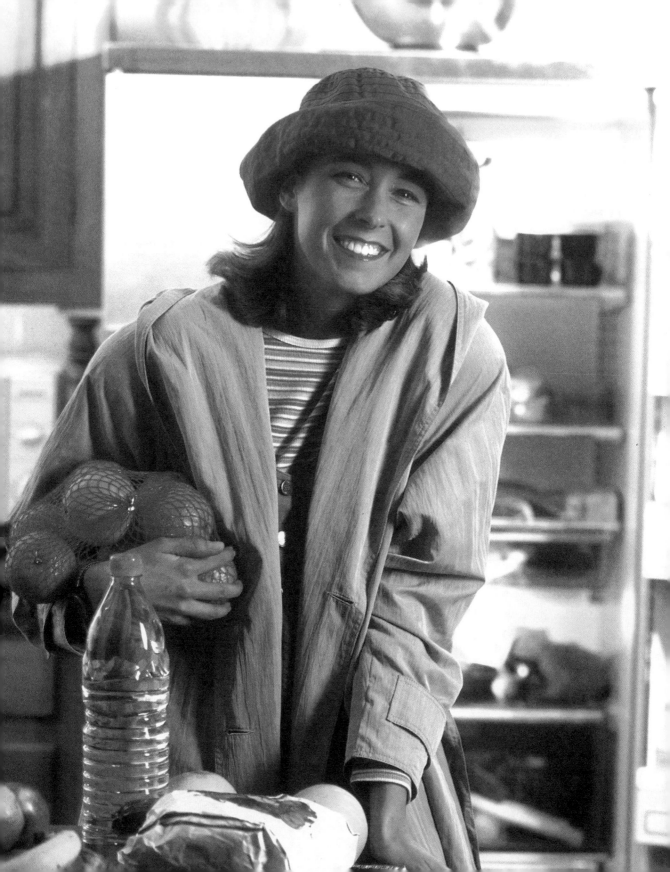

PART TWO

Remedies from Your Refrigerator

Slash your risk of all sorts of diseases just by putting the right foods on your dinner plate.

CHAPTER 3

The Seven Secrets of Healthy Living

You'll feel better and live longer if you adopt these seven strategies proven by scientific research.

When the USDA came up with its dietary guidelines for Americans, the researchers had the "average" person in mind. They knew that if they asked for too much, they had no hope for getting the average person to comply. The result: they didn't ask for much.

The truth is, following the USDA guidelines will improve your health if you're a couch potato who lives on Twinkies and hot dogs day in and day out. But if you already follow a relatively healthful lifestyle, the government's system won't lead you to optimum health.

That's why we consulted with many of the top researchers in the country to come up with the following new and improved set of dietary and lifestyle strategies. Follow our rules instead—and you're sure to achieve optimum health.

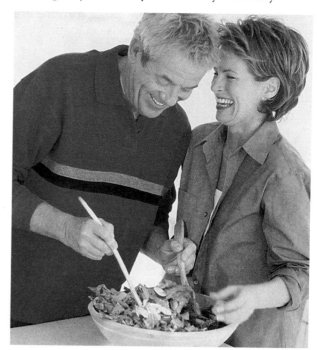

1. Eat tons of fruits and vegetables. We wish you could go to a cancer research conference and see all the scientists with lunch plates heaped with veggies and fruit. Eat nine servings a day.

2. Get more "good" fats. That means monounsaturated fats in olive oil, nuts, and peanut butter, and omega-3 fats in walnuts, canola oil, flaxseed, and fatty fish such as salmon. Avoid saturated fat (as in cheeseburgers!).

3. Cut way back on sugar. Every day, we eat an average of 21 teaspoons of added sugars. For starters, trade your soft drinks for iced tea, plain or sweetened with just a touch of honey.

4. Switch to whole grains. Evidence is mounting that we're eating far too much refined starch (white flour foods) for our own good. For example, women who eat mostly "white bread" diets have more breast cancer and diabetes.

5. If you drink alcohol, drink only a little. You know the rule about one drink a day for women, two drinks for men? Even that may be too much. One study of more than 40,000 adults found that people with the lowest risk of dying were women who averaged less than one drink per day and men who averaged less than two drinks per day.

6. Lose weight if you need to. Make this a huge health priority. Every extra pound puts you at greater risk of cancer, stroke, heart disease, diabetes, high blood pressure, and arthritis.

7. Do not sit around. Get 45 minutes of activity a day if you're trying to lose weight or keep it off. The exercise will not only burn calories but also help provide the motivation needed to stick to your healthful diet.

Eat Phytofoods and Feel the Difference!

Have you ever wondered if giving up processed foods would really be worth the effort? Instead, you'd munch on nuts, whole grains, fruits, and veggies—all packed with disease-fighting phytochemicals. Twelve women who did just that in the name of science reported an unexpected payoff: After just a few days on a phytofoods diet, they felt great.

First, the women were "forced" to eat a typical convenience-food diet for 4 weeks. Then they switched to phytofoods. After just 4 weeks of phytofoods, the women's total cholesterol dropped by 13 percent and their bad LDL cholesterol by 16 percent. The daily fiber boost (a total of 38 grams, up from a low of 15 grams) eliminated all traces of constipation, a possible risk factor for colon cancer.

But what impressed these women most? "They said that they felt so much better—lighter and with more energy—after only 1 week on phytofoods," says researcher Gene Spiller, Ph.D., of the SPHERA Foundation in Los Altos, California.

CHAPTER 4

Feel-Better Food

Eat to beat 20 common health problems, from allergies to vision loss.

Not so long ago, illness and disease were viewed as "things that just happen." Doctors considered them inevitable by-products of aging. It was never given much thought that what we ate—or didn't eat—could be a factor in our health.

Now we know better. Science and research have confirmed that as long as we have control over what food we put into our bodies, we'll have a good deal of control over our health. In the following pages, you'll see just how you can use food (plus herbs and supplements) as medicine. The wealth of vitamins, minerals, and other nutrients you'll be getting will help you prevent or treat just about every health condition you can think of, from allergies to vision problems.

‖ Allergies

You probably know the symptoms all too well: sneezing; nasal congestion; an itchy, runny nose; and red, watery eyes. The best solution is to avoid common allergy triggers altogether, but that's no small task. When symptoms leave you feeling miserable, you can fight back with these remedies.

Salt your nose. Using an over-the-counter saline nasal spray is a safe way of loosening mucus. To make your own salty solution, dissolve ½ teaspoon of salt in 8 ounces of lukewarm water. Then put it in a bulb syringe and flush it into your nose while leaning forward over the sink so that it can drip out. Use it daily. Look for bulb syringes at your local drugstore.

Learn to love licorice. This simple herbal medicine often produces dramatic results. Some herbalists recommend taking 250 to 500 milligrams of solid licorice (*Glycyrrhiza glabra*) twice a day continually for 3 months. Then take it every other day for an additional month, followed 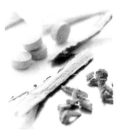 by every third day for a final month. Look for products made from the root of *Glycyrrhiza glabra*; avoid standardized and deglycyrrhizinated products.

‖ Anxiety

Too much anxiety can keep you up at night, bring on tension headaches, and leave you feeling restless, irritable, and downright exhausted. If anxiety is knocking at your door more often than you'd like, these herbal remedies can help you bid it a calm farewell.

Wind down with kava. Compared with drugs commonly prescribed for anxiety, the herb kava has shown similar results without all the side effects, says Susan B. Kowalsky, N.D., a naturopathic physician in Norwich, Vermont. When you buy kava capsules, look for a brand that is standardized to contain 30 percent kavalactones, the active ingredients in kava. Be sure to follow the label dosage instructions.

Soothe frazzled nerves with valerian. A popular anxiety remedy throughout Europe, valerian root can calm your nerves and help you sleep better, which can take the edge off your edginess. Research suggests that certain ingredients in valerian root—compounds called valepotriates and valeric acid—bind to the same brain receptors as the antianxiety drug diazepam (Valium). But valerian doesn't appear to cause the same bothersome side effects as diazepam—there's no grogginess or dependency. Experts suggest taking a 150-milligram capsule twice a day.

Inspect Your Chamomile

Chamomile tea is another herbal calmer. But take note: The chamomile flowers you use for a calming cup of tea should be yellow and white. If they're straw-colored, they're too old. Store chamomile in dark jars away from light and heat to prolong its healing properties.

‖ Asthma

Some people describe an asthma attack as a feeling similar to trying to breathe through a straw. The description fits perfectly, because during an attack, airways in the lungs squeeze shut, making it difficult to draw in air. At the same time, the narrowed airways become inflamed and filled with mucus, stifling the airways even further.

If you're already under medical care for your asthma, these two tips may further ease your symptoms.

Breathe better with ginkgo. "Ginkgo is a very good herb for asthma," says Shiva Barton, N.D., a licensed acupuncturist and lead naturopathic practitioner at Wellspace, a

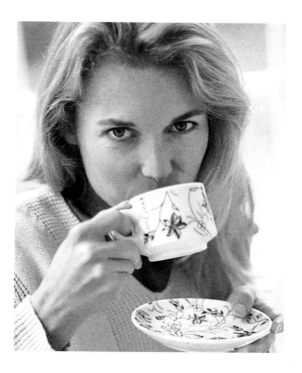

complementary health center in Cambridge, Massachusetts. "It works by relaxing the smooth muscle in the lungs and decreasing inflammation there."

Take one capsule two or three times a day and monitor your improvement during the next month or two, Dr. Barton suggests. If you experience positive results, reduce the dosage to the lowest amount that you need to feel well, she says.

Enjoy a cup of green tea. The same green tea that you enjoy so much with sushi or other Japanese food is also a good anti-inflammatory that helps control mucus secretion in asthma. You can drink it semiregularly over the long haul and daily when asthma symptoms are particularly bad. You can take green tea as supplements, but drinking tea made from the unfermented dried leaves makes more sense. You can find them loose or in tea bags in Japanese or Asian food stores; they're becoming more available in health food stores and grocery stores as well.

‖ Bad Breath

Bad breath occurs when you have too many odor-producing bacteria in your mouth, particularly on the back of your tongue. To stop them, try some of these time-honored tips.

Wet your whistle. Sip at least eight 8-ounce glasses of water daily. That'll keep your mouth moist, which is important because saliva helps wash away the food debris on which those noxious bacteria thrive. Swishing your mouth with water will also freshen your mouth after a meal.

Chew on some cardamom. Cardamom, a popular spice in Arabian cuisine, is rich in cineole, a potent antiseptic that kills bad-breath bacteria, says James A. Duke, Ph.D., author of *The Green Pharmacy Antiaging Prescriptions.*

You can buy whole cardamom in specialty herb shops and some supermarkets. To freshen bad breath, discard the pods and chew on some seeds, then discreetly spit them out.

Watch what you eat and drink. Try cutting back on coffee and alcohol, which dry your mouth. Also limit fatty foods and dairy products, which can change the acidity in your mouth so that it favors an overgrowth of odor-causing bacteria.

Canker Sores

These small, ulcerous sores sprout on the tender flesh of your inner cheek, lip, or tongue. They can turn orange or tomato juice into liquid fire or a slice of cheese pizza into a shard of glass. And brushing your teeth can become a truly bristling experience. Thankfully, canker sores heal on their own, usually within 2 weeks.

The following home remedies may help speed their disappearance.

Fight back with an echinacea tincture. This herb contains polysaccharides, substances that stimulate infection-fighting white blood cells. Apply the tincture to the sore three or four times a day.

Sip a cup of calendula tea. The petals of this cheery yellow flower have been used to heal sores and reduce inflammation, says Barry Sherr, a professional member of the American Herbalists Guild who practices in Danbury, Connecticut.

To make the tea, pour 1 cup of boiling water over 1 to 2 teaspoons of dried petals, steep for 10 to 15 minutes, and strain. Drink two cups of tea per day.

Cold Hands and Feet

Cold hands and feet can cause trouble when you want to snuggle with your sweetie on a chilly winter's night. Chronically cold extremities, on the other hand, can signal health problems. These may be related to menopause, an underactive thyroid gland, low iron levels, or sluggish circulation.

Since even healthy fingers and toes can turn frosty when winter sets in, try turning the heat up with these remedies that increase circulation and generate gentle warmth.

Brew some ginger tea. Ginger is known for its heat-generating abilities, and hot ginger tea is a delicious way to warm up. Put about 1 teaspoon of dried root in a small teapot and cover with 1 cup of boiling water. Steep for 10 minutes, then strain the tea into a mug and sweeten it with honey, if you like. Or try ginger capsules, which are widely available.

Warm up with cinnamon and cayenne. Cinnamon is a warming herb while cayenne increases circulation. Sprinkle a generous dusting of cinnamon on your morning oatmeal. Then make lunch a cayenne-spiced bowl of chili or stow some cayenne capsules in your day pack (follow the dosage directions on the label of the bottle you buy).

Cold Sores

Unsightly and annoying, cold sores—also called fever blisters—crop up around the edges of your lips, on the skin between your mouth and nose, and even inside your mouth. They're caused by the herpes simplex virus, which is transmitted by direct contact and can linger for years in nerve cells in your body, erupting occasionally. To help speed cold sore healing and soothe the accompanying pain and inflammation, try one or all of these remedies.

Soothe sores with echinacea. While no one compound is credited for its medicinal action, the herb *Echinacea angustifolia* is rich in polysaccharides, substances that have been found to stimulate infection-fighting white blood cells. Take 30 drops of the tincture in a glass of water three times a day.

Make a lemon balm rinse. Lemon balm contains tannins, antivirals that have been shown to hasten the healing of cold sores. Place 1 heaping tablespoon of the dried herb into 1 cup of boiling water and steep for 20 minutes. Let the tea cool, strain it, then swish it around in your mouth three to five times a day.

Dab it with myrrh. This fragrant, resinous herb works by directly attacking infectious invaders and by stimulating the body's nat-

ural defenses. Dab the tincture on the sore with a cotton swab up to 10 times a day.

Colds and Flu

A coworker sneezes, and a cloud of viruses fills the air. When one of those viruses takes hold of your body, you're in line for a nasty cold or flu. Research has found that some of the foods we eat every day contain powerful compounds that can help stop viruses from taking hold. And even when you're already sick, choosing the following foods will ease the discomfort and possibly even help you get better more quickly.

Eat more produce. Research shows that many fruits and vegetables contain a compound called glutathione, which stimulates the immune system to begin releasing large numbers of macrophages—specialized cells that seize viruses and mark them for destruction. Avocados, watermelons, asparagus, winter squash, and grapefruit are all rich in glutathione. Other good sources include okra, oranges, tomatoes, potatoes, cauliflower, broccoli, cantaloupe, strawberries, and peaches.

Maintain your C level. Another powerful compound in many fruits and vegetables is vitamin C, which lowers levels of histamine, a defensive chemical released by the immune system that causes stuffiness and other symptoms. Vitamin

Cold Hard Facts

When viruses attack, a strong immune system can churn out 10 million antibodies per hour to patrol your bloodstream and attack the enemy.

C may also strengthen white blood cells, which are essential for fighting infection. Get your C from fruit juices such as orange and cranberry.

Count on shades of orange and dark green. Some of the best foods for boosting immunity are those that contain beta-carotene, a plant pigment found in foods such as pumpkin, carrots, and mango. You can also get a lot of beta-carotene from leafy green vegetables such as spinach and kale.

Don't forget garlic. Garlic contains dozens of chemically active compounds, including allicin and alliin, which have been shown to kill germs directly. Garlic also appears to stimulate the immune system to release natural killer cells, destroying even more germs.

Drink more tea. Tea contains a compound called theophylline, which helps break up congestion. Tea also contains quercetin, a compound that may help prevent viruses from multiplying.

Zero in on zinc. Of all the minerals, zinc is probably the most important for keeping immunity strong. Too little zinc can lead to a drop in infection-fighting white blood cells, increasing your risk for getting sick. You can get zinc from wheat germ, Brazil nuts, and lean cuts of beef.

QUICK & HEALTHY
CARROT SOUP WITH LIME AND CHILES

This soup contains a wealth of cold-healing foods, from garlic to carrots to chicken broth.

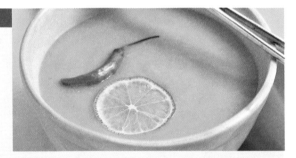

1	tablespoon olive or canola oil
1	large onion, finely chopped
2	large cloves garlic, chopped, or 1 tablespoon prepared chopped garlic
½	pound peeled, ready-to-eat baby carrots
½	cup uncooked instant brown rice
2	cans (14½ ounces each) fat-free, reduced-sodium chicken broth
1	cup water
½	teaspoon salt
2	tablespoons chopped green chiles
	Juice of 1 lime (about 2 tablespoons)

Heat the oil in a large nonstick saucepan over medium heat. Add the onion and sauté for 3 minutes. Add the garlic and sauté 1 minute longer.

Add the carrots, rice, broth, water, and salt to the saucepan. Bring to a boil, then reduce the heat to medium-low. Simmer, partially covered, for 20 minutes, or until the carrots are tender. Stir in the chiles and lime juice.

Puree the soup in a food processor or blender. The best way to puree this soup is to place half of the solids in the food processor and add just enough of the broth to liquefy the carrots and rice. Add the rest of the solids, then stir the puree back into the remaining broth. Reheat if necessary. Serve warm.

MAKES 4 SERVINGS (4 CUPS)
Per serving: 130 calories, 5 g protein, 21 g carbohydrates, 4 g fat, 0 mg cholesterol, 3 g dietary fiber, 717 mg sodium

Does Your Multi Have the Right Copper?

To fight the flu, look for multivitamin/mineral supplements that supply 100 percent of the Daily Value (DV) of immunity-boosting copper in the form of copper sulfate (also called cupric sulfate). Experts in copper absorption say that the type of copper used in most multivitamins, copper oxide (or cupric oxide), cannot be absorbed well by the human body. If your multi uses copper oxide, you won't be getting the copper insurance that your immune system may need. If the source of copper in your multi is not given, you can assume that the less expensive copper oxide was used.

Enhance immunity with yogurt. One study at the University of California, Davis, School of Medicine found that people who ate live-culture yogurt experienced a fourfold increase in immune-enhancing chemicals. Make sure that the yogurt label says "live cultures," and aim for a daily serving.

‖ Constipation

If your stools are usually small and hard, you find yourself having to strain, or 3 or more days pass between bowel movements, you're probably constipated. Here are some suggestions that can help get you "moving."

Drink like a fish. Many people are in chronic states of dehydration, says Theresa MacLean, N.D., R.Ph., a naturopathic physician and pharmacist based in Berwick, Nova Scotia. "When that happens, your bowels draw as much water as they can out of your food as it's being digested," Dr. MacLean explains. "This leaves the stool hard and

difficult to pass." Try to drink eight 8-ounce glasses of water a day.

Eat more rhubarb. These tart stalks ease constipation because they're a great source of fiber. When used properly (you should eat only the stalks, not the leaves, which can be toxic), rhubarb relieves constipation.

Use a "flaxative." If you take a fiber supplement to stay regular, you may want to give flaxseed a whirl. Just 2 tablespoons a day of this nutty-tasting seed offer enough insoluble fiber to keep you regular.

Consider an herbal stimulant. Cascara sagrada is probably the world's most popular laxative, says Dr. MacLean. The herb is even an ingredient in several over-the-counter constipation remedies. It contains anthraquinones, which stimulate the intestinal contractions that we recognize as nature's call. Take 15 to 20 drops of tincture once daily.

Note: Because cascara sagrada is such a powerful cathartic herb, it should not be used for more than 2 weeks at a time.

‖ natural WONDER

APPLE
Simply eating an apple a day can keep you regular. Apples are high in fiber and contain sugars that are hard for the body to digest. And what it can't digest, it pushes out.

‖ Depression

Some researchers suspect that what you eat can make a big difference in how you feel. For example, the following dietary strategies can help relieve depression by putting your brain chemicals back on an even keel.

Consume more carbs. Make sure that every meal contains some carbohydrate-rich foods, especially whole grain foods such as whole wheat bread, oatmeal, flaxseed, and brown rice. Carbohydrates trigger the release of insulin, which allows the amino acid tryptophan to freely enter your brain, causing serotonin levels to rise. And that serotonin boosts your mood.

Opt for omega-3s. Experts link low omega-3 consumption to increased rates of depression. Be sure to eat a rich source of omega-3 fats, such as fish, at least three times a week. The best fish for these "good" fats are salmon, mackerel, herring, and canned white tuna. (Two special omega-3 fats—called EPA and DHA—found in every fish are lacking in almost everyone's diet.) Other good sources of omega-3s include walnuts, walnut oil,

---

QUICK & HEALTHY

POACHED SALMON WITH TOASTED BREAD CRUMBS AND BASIL

The salmon in this recipe is loaded with mood-friendly omega-3 fatty acids.

2	teaspoons olive oil
¼	cup dried bread crumbs
1	tablespoon chopped pine nuts or other nuts
1	clove garlic, minced
1	tablespoon drained, chopped sun-dried tomatoes
2	tablespoons grated Parmesan cheese Salt and black pepper
2	tablespoons chopped fresh basil
4	salmon fillets, ½" thick and 4 ounces each, with skin

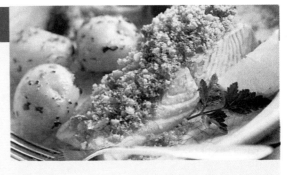

Simmer 4 cups of hot water in a 9" or 10" skillet over low heat.

Warm the oil in a smaller skillet on low heat. Add the bread crumbs and nuts and cook, stirring, for about 2 minutes, or until lightly toasted.

Add the garlic to the crumb mixture and cook, stirring, for 30 to 60 seconds longer, until the garlic is fragrant. Turn off the heat and stir in the tomatoes and cheese. Season with salt and pepper to taste, then stir in the basil.

Place the fillets skin side up in the simmering water, adding more hot water if needed to just cover. Cook for 10 minutes, or until just cooked through. Transfer to a platter, remove the skin by peeling it off from end to end, and discard.

Turn the fillets over, set on plates, and top with the bread crumb mixture.

MAKES 4 SERVINGS

Per serving: 263 calories, 25 g protein, 6 g carbohydrates, 12 g fat, 65 mg cholesterol, 0 g dietary fiber, 134 mg sodium

canola oil, ground flaxseed, flaxseed oil, or supplements. One supplement brand, Neuromins, uses DHA harvested from aquatic plants grown in tightly controlled conditions (fish actually get their omega-3s from eating the same kinds of plants). And since Neuromins uses plant sources of omega-3s, vegetarians can take them.

Make like Popeye. In one British study, researchers gave people with clinical depression 200 micrograms of folic acid (the supplement form of folate)—the amount in about ¾ cup of cooked spinach—or a placebo. After 1 year, those taking the folic acid felt their depression lift significantly, in some cases by as much as 40 percent.

Be sure to get Bs. Research has shown that vitamin B_6, found in fish, poultry, whole grains, and leafy greens, helps elevate serotonin to feel-good levels. Even though most people get plenty of B_6 in their diets, oral contraceptives or hormone-replacement therapy may lower B_6 levels.

| natural
WONDER
GREEN AND BLACK TEAS
Both green and black teas are high in tannins, which help your bowel form a protective film that prevents the absorption of toxins that cause diarrhea.

bark into 1 cup of hot water. Steep for 10 to 15 minutes, then strain. Use cinnamon this way only for short periods of time; chronic diarrhea requires medical attention.

Eat lightly. "The less food that your system has to process, the fewer symptoms of cramping and diarrhea you will experience," says Sheila Crowe, M.D., a gastroenterologist and assistant professor of medicine at the University of Texas Medical Branch at Galveston. If you're hungry, eat bland, light foods such as toast, cooked rice, or bananas.

Drink as much as you can. When you have diarrhea, your body loses water every time you go to the bathroom, so you can easily become dehydrated very quickly. Try to drink at least 10 glasses of clear liquid a day. You can also try chicken bouillon or a sports drink such as

‖ Diarrhea

Diarrhea is the body's way of saying, "Out with the bad"—a quick fix that will put your digestion back in balance. A sudden attack can originate from a number of sources, most commonly bacteria in food or water, a virus, or, more rarely, a parasite picked up while traveling abroad. But don't worry. Easing the pain and getting your bowel function back to normal is simple. Here's how.

Make cinnamon tea. Cinnamon is a natural astringent that will dry up your bowel. Mix 1 tablespoon of dried, powdered cinnamon

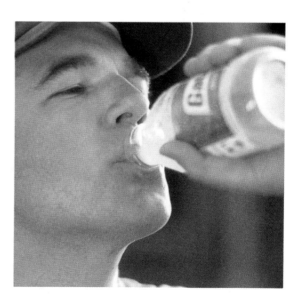

QUICK & HEALTHY

ASIAN-ACCENT CHICKEN AND BROCCOLI STIR-FRY

Thanks to the lean chicken breast, this recipe is high in protein and low in fat and carbohydrates—just what you need to fight fatigue.

1	**pound boneless, skinless chicken breasts, cut lengthwise into thin strips**
1	**tablespoon cornstarch**
2	**teaspoons brown sugar**
3	**tablespoons reduced-sodium soy sauce**
1	**tablespoon dry sherry (optional)**
2	**teaspoons dark Asian sesame oil**
1	**tablespoon corn oil or vegetable oil**
1	**teaspoon chopped fresh ginger**
4	**cups broccoli florets**
¼	**cup water or fat-free chicken broth**

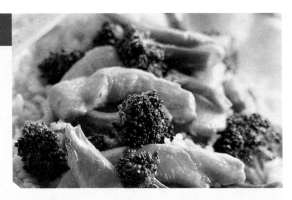

Place the chicken strips on a plate and dredge with the cornstarch and brown sugar. Sprinkle with the soy sauce, sherry (if using), and sesame oil. Toss well with 2 forks to coat strips evenly.

Place a wok or nonstick skillet on a burner over high heat. When the pan is hot, add 1 teaspoon of the corn oil. Turn the heat to medium-high, add the chicken, and cook until no longer pink and the juices run clear. Remove the chicken and set aside.

Lower the heat to medium. Add the remaining corn oil and ginger and stir for 30 seconds. Add the broccoli and cook, stirring constantly, for 2 minutes.

Add the chicken and water. Stir for 1 minute, or until the sauce is thickened. Remove from the heat. Serve with steaming-hot brown rice.

MAKES 4 SERVINGS

Per serving: 224 calories, 30 g protein, 10 g carbohydrates, 7.5 g fat, 66 mg cholesterol, 3 g dietary fiber, 545 mg sodium

Gatorade. These replace fluids as well as minerals and vitamins lost during an episode of diarrhea.

‖ Fatigue

You know the feeling. You go through the day in a daze, yearning for more sleep to help see you through to bedtime. You try to get by on coffee and sweet foods, which, ironically, are the worst things you can reach for when you're looking for extra energy. So what should you eat? Read on.

Get more protein. Our diets provide the raw materials needed to produce neurotransmitters—chemical messengers that play a role in regulating our energy levels. Studies have shown that changes in the levels of neurotransmitters such as dopamine and norepinephrine can dramatically affect energy levels, which is why they're sometimes called wake-up chemicals.

Tyrosine, an amino acid, is the building block for dopamine and norepinephrine. Tyrosine levels are elevated when you eat a high-protein food such as fish, chicken, or low-fat yogurt. Eating 3 to 4 ounces

Accuracy Counts

If you take your temperature orally while you're stuffy and breathing through your mouth, you could get an inaccurate reading. Instead, take it under your arm.

of a protein-rich food, such as broiled chicken breast or a hard-cooked egg, feeds your brain enough tyrosine to get the neurotransmitters flowing.

Watch the fat. Even though protein-rich foods can help boost energy, the fats that often come with them can drag you down. Digesting fats diverts blood from the brain, which can make you feel sluggish. So don't overload a turkey sandwich with high-fat cheese and mayonnaise; dress it with mustard, lettuce, and tomatoes instead.

Cut back on carbs. Eating food high in carbohydrates such as pasta and potatoes, especially for lunch, often leaves us nodding. Why? Because high-carbohydrate foods such as potatoes or rice cause the amino acid tryptophan to be delivered to the brain. This, in turn, jump-starts the production of serotonin, a "calm-down" chemical that regulates mood. What you want to do is bal-

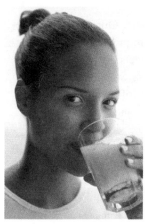

ance your carbohydrate/protein mix so that the bulk of your diet comes from complex carbohydrates, laced with a bit of proteins. Most people can improve their energy levels this way.

Drink orange juice. One study found that people who consumed at least 400 milligrams of vitamin C a day reported feeling less fatigued than those consuming less than 100 milligrams. In both cases the amount of vitamin C was considerably higher than the Daily Value (DV) of 60 milligrams. To boost your intake, reach for foods high in vitamin C such as orange juice, strawberries, cantaloupe, red bell peppers, and broccoli.

Get your iron. Iron is also essential for energy. This is particularly true for women, who can lose large amounts of iron during menstruation. Even small iron deficiencies can leave you weary. Fortunately, iron is very easy to get by eating quick-cooking Cream of Wheat and lean red meats.

‖ Fever

Besides the above-average temperature, typical symptoms of fever include chills, sweating, headache, dry mouth, muscle aches, fatigue, and sleepiness. Experts say that you should treat a fever only if it makes you feel uncomfortable. Here are some self-care tips to help you start feeling better in no time.

Drink up. "Drinking fluids is important when treating a fever—especially if you're sweating—in order to prevent dehydration," says Pamela Tucker, M.D., assistant professor of medicine in the division of infectious diseases at Johns Hopkins University School of Medicine in Baltimore. "Aim for eight glasses of liquids a day. Drink water, but drink orange juice and other fruit juices high in vitamin C, too." Research suggests that vitamin C may help boost your immune system by preventing the formation of free radicals—substances in your body that weaken the immune system.

Try a sports or soft drink. You can also drink sports drinks and regular (but not diet) soft drinks, says Susan Black, M.D., a board member of the American Academy of Family Physicians. "When you have a fever, your body's metabolism is speeded up, and you burn extra calories," she notes. "Skip the diet sodas until your fever breaks; your body needs calories."

‖ Flatulence

Although it's a completely normal bodily function, passing gas can be downright embarrassing. The culprit, most likely, is in what you eat. Try these tactics for keeping gas to a minimum.

De-gas the beans. Indigestible sugars in beans are notorious gas producers. If you elect to keep high-fiber beans in your diet, help is at hand. Before you cook them, soak dry beans overnight in a potful of water with a couple of tablespoons of vinegar. That will help reduce gassiness.

Savor Every Morsel

The more slowly you eat, the less air you swallow, so the less likely you are to suffer from gas.

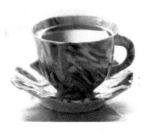

Drink peppermint tea. Peppermint is one of the oldest known remedies for gas, says James S. Sensenig, N.D., distinguished visiting professor at the University of Bridgeport College of Naturopathic Medicine in Connecticut. Pick up some peppermint tea at a grocery or health food store. (Just check the label to be sure it's herbal, not flavored, tea.) If you have a bunch of peppermint, add 1 cup of boiling water to ¼ to ½ cup of fresh, clean leaves. Steep for 10 minutes, then strain out the herb. Sip the tea slowly after it has cooled a little.

Try acidophilus. Acidophilus bacteria are friendly microorganisms that live in your intestines and support good digestion. If you suffer from excess gas, eat a serving of yogurt daily—make sure it contains live cultures—or buy acidophilus capsules, which you'll find refrigerated at the health food store. Follow label directions for proper dosage.

‖ Headaches

We all know how miserable a headache can make you feel. Tension headaches, the most common type, may be related to stress and tension. Migraine headaches, on the other hand, may start as an electrical change in the brain, followed by a disturbed bloodflow to the head, causing pain. Luckily, many kinds of headaches respond to simple measures. So if your doctor has ruled out a medical reason for your headaches, give these at-home remedies a try.

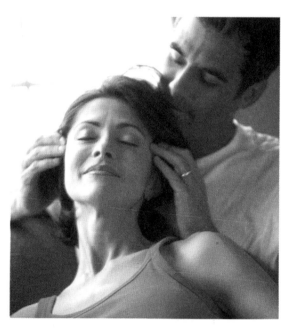

Massage with oils of lavender and peppermint. Lavender and peppermint essential oils can be used individually to relieve a tension headache, but when blended, they are more effective, says Connie Catellani, M.D., medical director of the Miro Center for Integrative Medicine in Evanston, Illinois. To make a headache oil, mix 1 tablespoon of vegetable oil, 10 drops of lavender essential oil, 5 drops of peppermint essential oil, and the contents of a vitamin E capsule in an amber glass bottle, then shake well. Massage into your temples, the back of your neck, or wherever you feel tension.

Take a coffee break. "If you feel a migraine coming on, have a strong cup of coffee. Then take aspirin or ibuprofen according to package instructions," says Patricia Solbach, Ph.D., director of the Center for Clinical Research at the Menninger Clinic in Topeka, Kansas. Caffeine acts as a vasoconstrictor, which helps migraines.

Try feverfew. The herb feverfew prevents migraines, but it's not useful for treating a headache once it starts. Every morning, take one 300-milligram tablet to head off the pain.

‖ Heartburn

Any number of things can bring on a case of heartburn: eating spicy foods, smoking cigarettes, drinking alcohol, being severely overweight, or just lying down or bending over right after a meal. For most of us, certain simple dietary and lifestyle changes will cool the burn and keep food in our stomachs where it belongs. Among the strategies that experts recommend are the following:

Fast before sleeping. "Try not to eat or drink anything for 2 to 3 hours before you go to bed," says Robyn Karlstadt, M.D., a gastroenterologist at Wyeth-Ayerst Pharmaceuticals in Philadelphia. That way, all your food will empty from your stomach before you go to bed.

Chew some gum. For temporary relief of heartburn, try chewing gum. "It stimulates the flow of saliva, which neutralizes acid and helps push digestive juices back down where they belong," says Tim McCashland, M.D., associate professor of medicine in the department of gastroenterology at the University of Nebraska Medical Center in Omaha.

Speed digestion with turmeric. Bitter herbs help stimulate the flow of digestive juices, moving food along and preventing acid buildup. Spice up your food with the bitter herb turmeric. If flavoring your food isn't enough, take two or three turmeric capsules (½ to 1 gram), available at health food stores, before a meal.

‖ Memory Problems

What we sometimes assume is the onset of "senility" may actually be caused by marginal nutritional deficiencies. When we run low on certain nutrients, our mental performance dips. These deficiencies become more common as we get older and our bodies are less efficient at absorbing certain vitamins, minerals, and other vital compounds.

By getting enough of key brain-boosting nutrients and adopting other lifestyle strategies, like those recommended here, you can keep your mind sharp for a lifetime.

Fill your plate with pastas, breads, and cereals. The B vitamins are perhaps the most essential nutrients for maintaining mental function. Your body uses B vitamins to turn food into mental energy and to manufacture and repair your brain tissue. The easiest way to make sure you get enough brain-boosting B vitamins is to eat enriched grain products. Other good sources of B vitamins include pork tenderloin,

---

QUICK & HEALTHY
MEDITERRANEAN PASTA

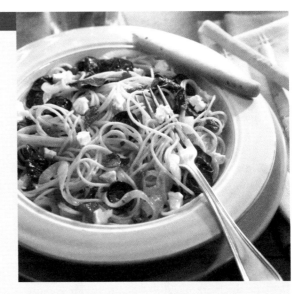

Pasta is high in B vitamins that help keep brain tissue healthy.

½	**cup sun-dried tomatoes**
8	**ounces angel hair pasta**
1	**tablespoon olive oil**
2	**onions, chopped**
1	**teaspoon dried oregano**
1	**package (10 ounces) fresh spinach, chopped, or 2 packages (9 ounces) frozen chopped spinach, thawed and squeezed dry**
2	**tablespoons chopped pitted kalamata olives or black olives**
1	**cup (5 ounces) crumbled feta cheese**

Soak the tomatoes in hot water for 10 minutes. Drain and chop.

Cook the pasta per package directions.

Warm the oil in a large nonstick skillet over medium heat. Add the onions and oregano. Cook for 10 minutes, or until the onions are tender.

Add the spinach, cover, and cook for 5 minutes, or until the spinach is wilted. Add the olives, tomatoes, and pasta. Toss to mix. Sprinkle with the cheese.

MAKES 4 SERVINGS

Per serving: 471 calories, 19 g protein, 59 g carbohydrates, 19 g fat, 50 mg cholesterol, 5 g dietary fiber, 908 mg sodium

chicken breast, turkey, lean ground beef, steamed clams, baked potatoes, bananas, and chickpeas.

Eat lots of produce. Fruits and vegetables are packed with antioxidants, compounds that block the effects of harmful oxygen molecules called free radicals. Scientists think that these abundant antioxidants, especially the flavonoids in spinach and blueberries, may reduce inflammation, a process that may impair brain tissue as we age. Produce is also rich in boron, a mineral that may help keep your mind sharp. In tests of memory, perception, and attention, people low in boron did not perform as well as when they had higher amounts. And a current study found that reflexes and mental alertness improved when people were given additional boron.

Drink more water. Not getting enough water can cause the mind to get fuzzy. One of the symptoms of severe dehydration is mental confusion.

Enjoy coffee—in moderation. While caffeine has been shown to improve memory, for some people, the after-coffee slump can result in mental fogginess.

‖ Stress

Late for work—grab a doughnut. The report's due—pour another cup of coffee. The children are yelling—take an ice cream break. Stress is all around us, and food often provides a welcome, if momentary, break. Unfortunately, the foods we often turn to in times of stress, like coffee and sweets, have a way of making us feel even more frazzled later on.

It doesn't have to be this way. Research has shown that eating more of some foods and less of others can cause stress hormones to decline. Making slight dietary changes will produce physical changes in the brain that can make the world's problems a little bit easier to handle.

Calm down with carbohydrates. Mashed potatoes. Fresh-baked bread. A steaming plate of pasta. These are just a few of the "comfort foods" that many of us instinctively turn to in times of stress. As it turns out, our instincts are dead-on. Researchers have found that foods high in carbohydrates produce changes in the brain that can take the edge off stress.

Cut back on caffeine. Researchers at the University of Minnesota in Morris found that half of the nearly 300 people in their study drank more coffee or caffeine-containing soft drinks during high-pressure times. Caffeine produces a quick zing that can momentarily make you feel more relaxed and confident. Fairly quickly, however, it stimulates the production of cortisol, a stress hormone that raises blood pressure and heart rate. This can make you feel more stressed than you did before.

Munch on a banana. Research suggests that foods high in vitamin B_6, such as bananas, potatoes, and prunes, can relieve irritability and stress, making people feel just a little bit better. One banana gives you 0.7 milligram of the 2 milligrams a day of B_6 that you need.

‖ Stomachache

We use the word *stomachache* as a catchall term for a variety of belly discomforts, including knots, a dull ache, an acidy feeling, cramps, or even nausea. The next time you encounter these symptoms, try over-the-counter acid suppressors and antacids, or give these remedies a shot. (If you experience recurrent stomachaches, make sure you see your doctor.)

Sip a soothing tea. For chronic stomach ailments, drinking chamomile tea regularly for more than 2 months may help relieve even obstinate digestive problems. Steep 1 tablespoon of chamomile or two chamomile tea bags in 1 cup of boiling water, and drink three times a day, before meals. Continue for at least a year to ensure remission.

Adopt the BRAT diet. As your stomach feels better, you'll have more of an appetite, but the best way to make sure the ache is banished for good is to stick to a BRAT (bananas, rice, applesauce, and dry toast) diet. Even on the BRAT plan, you should eat very little and add each new food gradually so that your cranky stomach won't have to work too hard to digest it. Once you feel entirely better, then you can go back to normal eating.

Reach for dried blueberries. Dried blueberries have been shown to be absorbent and to inhibit bacterial adhesion, thus reducing infection. "There is a long history of using dried blueberries for diarrhea and upset stomach," says Mary Ellen Camire, Ph.D., associate professor in the department of food science and human nutrition at the University of Maine in Orono. Try up to 3 tablespoons of dried blueberries. Don't use fresh or frozen berries, however, because the moisture in fresh or frozen fruit may cause diarrhea.

| natural
WONDER
ROSEMARY TEA
A staple in any spice rack, rosemary contains volatile oils that taste bitter. These bitters stimulate the flow of digestive juices, while other compounds in rosemary actually calm stomach spasms.

‖ Vision Problems

Most of us enjoy a colorful sunset or an ocean vista without giving much thought to the miracle

Have Some Fat with That

For the lutein in your spinach to prevent vision loss, you must eat it along with some fat. In one study, researchers found that getting lutein with just a teaspoon of fat raised blood lutein levels by 88 percent in 14 people. "Without fat, we know that lutein absorption is negligible," says nutrition researcher Cheryl Rock, Ph.D., of the University of California, San Diego. Dr. Rock's favorite recipe to make sure she absorbs her lutein? It's easy: Just toss 2 cups of raw spinach with 1 tablespoon of walnut oil, 1 teaspoon of mustard, and 3 tablespoons of balsamic vinegar. *Prevention* testers loved this dressing!

I DID IT!

Oz Garcia: He Thought It Was a Long Shot, but He Was Wrong

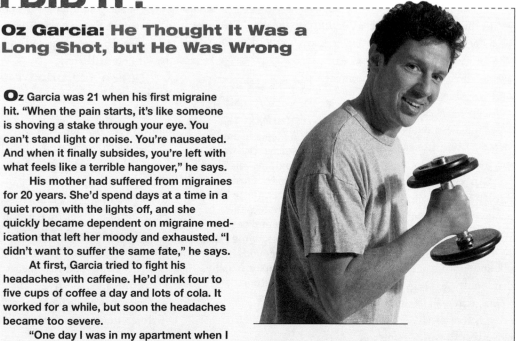

Oz Garcia was 21 when his first migraine hit. "When the pain starts, it's like someone is shoving a stake through your eye. You can't stand light or noise. You're nauseated. And when it finally subsides, you're left with what feels like a terrible hangover," he says.

His mother had suffered from migraines for 20 years. She'd spend days at a time in a quiet room with the lights off, and she quickly became dependent on migraine medication that left her moody and exhausted. "I didn't want to suffer the same fate," he says.

At first, Garcia tried to fight his headaches with caffeine. He'd drink four to five cups of coffee a day and lots of cola. It worked for a while, but soon the headaches became too severe.

"One day I was in my apartment when I felt another one coming on. For lack of anything better, I opened a book on fasting, which a friend had left behind. I was grasping at straws but decided to give it a shot," he says. Garcia ate nothing all day and drank only water. When he woke in the morning, his headache was gone.

"That book became my bible. I read it over and over; the more I read, the more I began to think my diet might be affecting my health," he says. Garcia soon gave up coffee. "Almost immediately, a headache started, but I didn't give in. I had to find out if this was the road to a cure," he says. "The pain raged for days, and then, as if by magic, it stopped. I awoke one morning feeling better than ever. I was alert and rested, and my head felt fine."

He then became mostly vegetarian. And he threw away his cigarettes.

Garcia bought running shoes and started running/walking the 1.6-mile loop around the reservoir in New York City's Central Park. Gradually, over the course of a few weeks, he added a second lap. Within a few months, he was running the entire park, a 6-mile loop. In 1979, he ran his first marathon.

"With each change, I felt better. My headaches became fewer and further apart. My sleeping improved, and I was more alert. My stomach stopped hurting, and my mood became more upbeat. Even my skin and sinuses cleared, and my gums stopped bleeding," he says.

"Today, I'm happier than ever. At 47, I run 3 to 4 miles most mornings, more on weekends. I do upper-body strength training a couple times a week and stick to a low-fat diet. I now eat some chicken and fish, and while I occasionally have a cup of coffee at Sunday brunch or eat steak once or twice a year, I'll never return to my old ways."

of vision. But over time, the ravages of sunlight, smoking, age, and poor eating habits start to take their toll. And for people with eye diseases—such as cataracts and age-related macular degeneration (ARMD)—the loss of vision can be profound.

The specific fruits and veggies mentioned here contain a variety of protective compounds that can stop damage to the eyes before problems get a foothold.

QUICK & HEALTHY
SPECTACULAR SPINACH

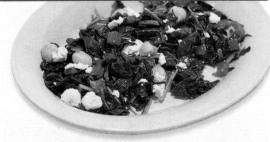

To consume more lutein-rich spinach, try this recipe.

2	packages (9 ounces each) frozen spinach
½	cup chickpeas, rinsed
½	cup crumbled feta cheese
1	ounce sliced pimientos

Heat and drain the spinach, then mix in the chickpeas, cheese, and pimientos.

MAKES 5 SERVINGS (2½ CUPS)

Per serving: 80 calories, 4.2 g protein, 8.4 g carbohydrates, 2.5 g fat, 1.6 mg cholesterol, 3.5 g dietary fiber, 456 mg sodium

Add spinach to the menu. Eating dark green leafy vegetables such as spinach is absolutely the best way to prevent ARMD. Lutein, abundant in spinach, shows promise against ARMD. Lutein protects the retina by absorbing damaging blue light, and its antioxidant power resists damage from any light that does get through. One study has shown that spinach can improve night vision, contrast, and adjustment to bright lights as well as vision distortions. Eat at least ½ cup, four to seven times a week. Enjoy other lutein-rich foods such as kale, collards, or turnip greens, and choose fresh, frozen, or canned.

Enjoy your apricots and carrots. Every time light passes through the eyes, it triggers the release of tissue-damaging free radicals. Left unchecked, these destructive oxygen molecules attack and damage the lenses of the eyes, possibly setting the stage for cataracts. To fight this, you need the beta-carotene in apricots and carrots that the body converts to vitamin A, which helps protect your eyes.

Prevent problems with pumpkin. A rich source of beta-carotene, pumpkin—especially canned pumpkin—also contains carotenoids lutein and zeaxanthin, which are found in the lenses of the eyes. Studies suggest that eating foods high in these compounds may help block the formation of cataracts and ARMD.

Don't overlook fish. A study of 2,900 people found that those who ate fish once or more a month had half the risk of developing ARMD compared with those who ate fish less often. Scientists think that seafood's omega-3 fats—also found in the retina—may protect against the disease.

Aging Alert

Learn about the latest breakthrough in nutrition research: superfoods that can stop aging in its tracks.

An average of three times a day, every day, you get the opportunity to protect your body from the effects of aging. Over the course of a single year, that's more than 1,000 individual chances to boost your immunity and reverse disease.

Every bite of broccoli or apple, every spoonful of whole grain cereal, every sip of water or fat-free milk, every taste of tuna fish or tofu is a contributor to your health and a protector of your youth. While we don't often think of food as having magic bullets in the sense that miracle drugs are magic bullets, they really do produce miraculous amounts of prevention, protection, and healing in our bodies.

Some foods protect us by boosting immunity. Others sweep out the digestive tract and keep it in top-notch working order. Still others can help reduce the risk of cancer, protect us from heart attack, maintain brainpower by deterring stroke and memory loss, strengthen our bones, and guard our vision.

The net result of all this good eating? A younger you. That's because food is not just a builder, it is also a protector. And if you eat the antiaging foods recommended by leading doctors, nutritionists, and dietitians, you are truly using the best tactic there is to protect yourself from aging.

Remember the "Four Food Groups" you learned way back in elementary school? When it comes to antiaging foods, the most important food groups for you to focus on are the high-fiber food group, the high-protein group, and the high-antioxidant group. Here's what you need to know about each.

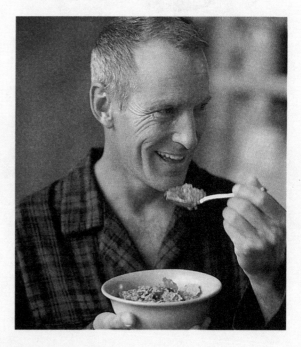

High-Fiber Foods

"If fiber were a nutrient, it would be one of the most deficient in American diets," says Cathy Kapica, R.D., Ph.D., assistant professor of nutrition and clinical dietetics at Finch University of Health Sciences/The Chicago Medical School. Fiber, often called bulk, is just the indigestible portion of plant foods. Because it is indigestible, it travels through your intestines without being absorbed by your body. This seemingly useless attribute is precisely what makes it such a wonderful disease preventer.

All plant foods generally have two kinds of dietary fiber: soluble and insoluble. But some fruits, grains, and vegetables are better sources of one kind than the other. Soluble fiber, particularly abundant in oats and dried beans, dissolves in the watery contents of the gastrointestinal tract to form a gel. This gel corrals some of the fats, cholesterol, and chemicals in the intestinal tract that would otherwise get absorbed. For example, soluble fiber is great for doing a sweep-up of bile acids, which your body makes from cholesterol and uses to break down fats in your small intestine. Soluble fiber helps carry bile out of the body and can aid in lowering your overall blood cholesterol level.

But insoluble fiber, particularly abundant in bran cereals, seems the more important fiber when it comes to keeping the colon cancer-free. It works like a sponge, soaking up water in the intestinal tract. Since the spongelike effect makes intestinal wastes much heavier, they move faster through the intestinal tract. "Not only does this keep you more regular, it also may help prevent colon cancer," says Dr. Kapica. Besides ushering out potentially cancer-causing substances, insol-

Top 20 Antiaging Foods

This top 20 list is literally the best of the best—the 20 foods that have unquestionable star-quality when it comes to body and mind protection.

1. Spinach
2. Fat-free milk
3. Wheat germ
4. Canned pink salmon with bones
5. Kidney beans
6. Papaya
7. Black-eyed peas
8. Canned tuna
9. Broccoli
10. Acorn squash
11. Tofu
12. Bulgur wheat
13. Whole wheat bread
14. Sweet potatoes
15. Swiss chard
16. Fat-free yogurt, plain
17. Bok choy
18. Tomatoes
19. Cantaloupe
20. Sunflower seeds

uble fiber also cuts down on the number of polyps that form in the gastrointestinal tract. And that's an important service because polyps are small, sometimes precancerous growths that may grow larger if left alone.

Vegetables and whole grain foods are your best sources of fiber. When it comes to eating your vegetables, broccoli is one mean green you should indulge in as often as possible. It protects both your heart and your digestive system. "Broccoli really might be the ultimate vegetable," says Robert E. C. Wildman, R.D., Ph.D., professor of nutrition and dietetics at the University of Delaware in Newark.

Broccoli's deep green color signals the presence of plenty of beta-carotene. This precursor to vitamin A is known as an antioxidant. In the body, antioxidants put the brakes on molecules called free radicals, tough guys who wander about causing invisible damage that eventually leads to aging and increased risk for chronic diseases like cancer.

In addition to its vitamin content, broccoli boasts at least four kinds of phytochemicals, cancer fighters in food that are neither vitamins nor minerals. With names like sulforaphane, phenethyl isothiocyanate, monoterpene, and indole, you might not believe that these are natural ingredients. But in fact, these tongue-twisting, health-enhancing compounds are abundant in nature.

Here are some tips on how you can get more broccoli in your meals every day. These recommendations come from Linda Nebeling, R.D., Ph.D., a nutritionist for the Five a Day for Better Health program at the National Cancer Institute in Bethesda, Maryland.

Eat it plain or with a dip. Raw or lightly steamed broccoli has a hearty, satisfying crunch. When dunked into a low-fat dip, this veggie makes a great alternative to chips.

Don't forget about soup. Broccoli doesn't have to be relegated to the corner of your dinner plate. Bring it to center stage by letting it star in a pot of soup. Cream of broccoli soup is a whole different way to capitalize on this vegetable. Substitute fat-free evaporated milk for

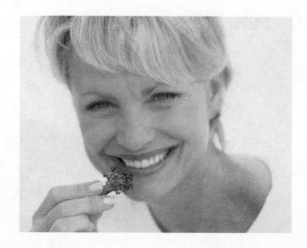

heavy cream and use a blender to puree cooked broccoli until it's smooth.

Pick some florets. If preparing broccoli seems like a chore, check out the packages of already-trimmed broccoli at your grocery store. Florets, the top part of the vegetable with the thick stems already removed, are just right for steaming or sautéing.

High-Protein Foods

Quality protein is key to good immune system function as you age, and good immunity means less cancer, heart disease, and other age-related diseases. "Fortunately, Americans generally do eat enough protein," says Dr. Kapica. As we age and the nest empties, however, we are less likely to fix complete meals. "Relying on salads, soups, and toast often means coming up short on protein," she notes. Look to fish, lean meat, fat-free milk, and legumes for protein.

Seafood is a great low-fat, protein-rich alternative to red meat, says Dr. Wildman. But there are

Foods to Flee From

While you're filling up on antiaging superfoods, it's also important to steer clear of foods that can undermine your good intentions. These are the ones that offer nil in the way of nutrition, while serving up ferocious amounts of fat and cholesterol. If you occasionally indulge in small amounts, these foods won't do much damage. Just be sure they don't make it to your high-rotation list.

Here are some of the worst offenders, say Robert E. C. Wildman, R.D., Ph.D., professor of nutrition and dietetics at the University of Delaware in Newark, and other experts.

Canned meat products. Canned convenience meat made its first appearance on dinner plates during World War II. Innocent-looking enough, the oftentimes pink pork product can contain 24 grams of fat in every little 3-ounce serving—nearly the amount found in two ground-beef burgers.

Fettucine Alfredo. Also known as heart attack on a plate, just one serving of this rich, cream-and-cheese-based Italian dish contains 857 calories, 54 grams of fat, and 250 milligrams of cholesterol. And that doesn't include the garlic bread that often goes with it. It's saturated fat all the way—so do your best to keep away.

Pound cake. Ever wonder why it's called pound cake? The name refers to the pound of butter traditionally included in this devil of a dessert. This high-calorie choice will fill your arteries with 44 milligrams of cholesterol per slice. Better bet: Forgo the pound cake (and the pounds) and opt for practically fat-free angel food cake.

Premium ice cream. There's nothing like a cool ice cream sundae on a hot summer afternoon. Nothing worse for your waistline is more like it. "The sugar and the fat in ice cream work really well together to make you gain weight," says Diane Grabowski-Nepa, R.D., nutrition educator at the Pritikin Longevity Center in Santa Monica, California. "And it's simply much too easy to overdo when it comes to portion size." She recommends low-fat or fat-free frozen yogurt as a stand-in.

Spareribs. This all-American meat is too high in fat to justify including in any healthy diet. With nearly 26 grams of fat per 3-ounce serving, a double helping of spareribs could easily fill an entire day's fat budget. And with 103 milligrams of cholesterol and high levels of saturated fat, your heart will thank you for sparing the spareribs.

Specialty coffees. Beware of gourmet cappuccinos and mochaccinos made with full-fat milk. According to Ted Lingle, executive director of the Specialty Coffee Association of America, the difference between a 12-ounce whole-milk cappuccino and the fat-free version is as much as 5 grams of fat. So, if you yearn for latte, be sure to specify the skinny variety. And you won't even notice a difference. Fat-free milk froths up just as nicely as the full-fat stuff, says Lingle.

even more benefits to be found in the omega-3-rich "fatty fish" that thrive in the deepest, coldest ocean waters. For boosting immunity, both tuna fish and pink salmon (with bones) are high on the super-food list because both have plenty of protein, selenium, and the all-important B vitamins in addition to their body-friendly fish oil. Fortunately for those on the go, tuna and salmon are quick and easy to prepare. Here are some suggestions to get more in your diet.

Open a can. Canned tuna and canned salmon are convenient and inexpensive, notes Diane Grabowski-Nepa, R.D., nutrition educator at the Pritikin Longevity Center in Santa Monica, California. To be sure that you're getting the most omega-3 fatty acids possible, choose water-packed seafood, she advises. That's because fatty acids tend to dissolve in vegetable oils. And if the fish is packed in oil, you will lose the fatty acids when you pour out the oil.

Try seafood Italiano. Canned tuna or salmon isn't just for lunch-box sandwiches. This seafood lends itself nicely to many other dishes. Try adding a can of either one to marinara sauce and toss with linguine.

Have some easy sea salad. Mix a can of tuna or salmon with hard-cooked egg whites, boiled small potatoes, and steamed green beans. Drizzle with vinegar and olive oil. In just minutes, you'll have an impromptu niçoise salad.

The Super Fluid

In a world of celebrity-sponsored soft drinks, microbrewed beers, super-hyped sports beverages, and gourmet-flavored coffees, plain water often gets relegated to last choice. And that's too bad, according to Nancy Clark, R.D., director of nutrition services at SportsMedicine Brookline in Brookline, Massachusetts, and author of *Nancy Clark's Sports Nutrition Guidebook, Second Edition.* "Water," she says, "is the ultimate nutrient."

Water is essential to human health. It's possible to survive for weeks without food, but you'll only last a few days without water. Because our bodies are anywhere from 60 to 70 percent water, a shortage can quickly turn into a crisis. Severe dehydration can lead to life-threatening heart disturbances. But even mild dehydration can cause dizziness, fatigue, cramps, and nausea. And for overall digestive health, it's essential as well since you always need the liquid to bulk up soluble and insoluble fiber.

The standard recommendation is at least eight glasses (that's 8 ounces, or 1 cup, each) of water a day for the average adult, says Clark. Of course, no one's average. Depending on your gender, your weight, your age, your activity level, and the temperature outside, your body's need for fresh water can be even higher.

You can tell how you're doing in the drinking department by monitoring your urine. "Urine should be practically clear," says Clark. "And there should be a good volume of it, too." In other words, if you are not visiting the rest room every 2 to 4 hours, you probably need to drink more.

A Step beyond Vegetarianism

It's not difficult to see that fruits and vegetables are many of the superfoods that help protect your body from age-related disease and health problems. So you may be asking yourself about the benefits of becoming a vegetarian.

People on the most strict vegetarian diet—called a vegan diet—don't eat any animal products, including meat, fish, eggs, and cheese. The payoff for following this pared-down diet comes in the form of some impressive health benefits, says Reed Mangels, R.D., Ph.D., nutrition advisor for the Vegetarian Resource Group in Baltimore. Vegans have a low risk for many diseases including diabetes, heart disease, and some forms of cancer. "People theorize lots of reasons why that's so," she says. "Vegans generally get more fiber, more phytochemicals from the vegetables they eat, and fewer pesticides."

The key to vegan eating lies in enjoying a variety of foods. It's very important to choose foods from a range of sources—and that's not only to keep you healthy but also to avoid boredom. Just as no one could live on a regimen of double cheeseburgers, a diet consisting solely of broccoli and brussels sprouts will also be less than optimal.

High-Antioxidant Foods

Your brain needs oxygen to function well, and it receives more oxygen when your arteries are clear. Antioxidants are one of your best defenses against artery-clogging plaque buildup.

Swiss researchers have turned up evidence that people with the highest blood levels of the antioxidants vitamin C and beta-carotene score higher on memory tests. Most of the study participants with the highest blood levels of the nutrients got them from eating real food, not from taking supplements.

While research teams are still thinking through why antioxidant foods keep them thinking clearly, they hypothesize that antioxidant nutrients or something else in antioxidant-containing foods may protect fragile brain cells from oxidative damage. This type of damage can break down neurons, which can keep them from properly transferring signals that translate into thinking. Of course, antioxidant nutrients may also keep blood vessels clear so that oxygen-rich blood can flow at full force to the brain cells—also necessary to keep them working their best.

The most important antioxidants seem to be the carotenes found in brightly colored fruits and vegetables, vitamin C found abundantly in citrus fruits, and vitamin E, which is tougher to come by in the food world. Nuts, wheat germ, and olive oil are your best vitamin E sources. But you should consider supplementing with up to 400 IU of vitamin E a day to ensure that you're getting enough of this important nutrient.

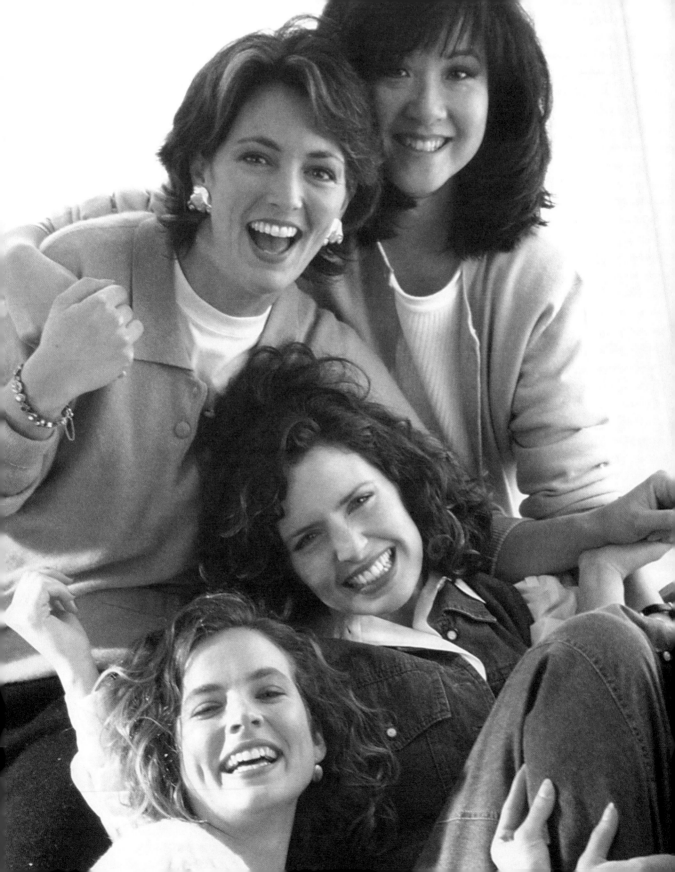

PART THREE

For Women Only

A woman's body is different from a man's—and so are her nutritional needs. Discover the dietary strategies that can keep you feeling and looking your best.

CHAPTER 5

Made Just for You

These are the supplements that no woman should be without.

First christened "growth factors" in 1906, vitamins and minerals are turning out to be critical elements in overall health. At one time, nutritionists said that few women needed supplements of any kind. They've changed their tune.

"Most of the nutrition experts I know take supplements," says Gordon M. Wardlaw, R.D., Ph.D., associate professor of medical dietetics at Ohio State University in Columbus.

Try as they might, even nutritionists find it tough to figure out how to cover all of their nutritional bases simply by eating a healthful diet.

If they can't do it, how are we supposed to manage? That's why women need supplements. Here, you'll discover nutrients every woman needs and how to get them, based on the latest findings about these substances.

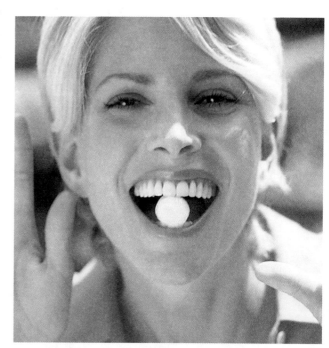

‖ Vitamin C

One overview article found that women getting 300 milligrams of vitamin C a day—the equivalent of about 4½ oranges or 3 cups of orange juice—had 30 percent less breast cancer risk than women who got less vitamin C.

Another study showed that women who took vitamin C supplements for at least 10 years were 77 percent less likely to develop cataracts than women who received the vitamin only through their diets. Vitamin C also plays a role in bone protection.

Best food sources: Go for pineapple, broccoli, peppers, cantaloupe, strawberries, oranges, kiwifruit, and pink grapefruit.

How much to aim for: The Daily Value for vitamin C is 60 milligrams a day. But vitamin C guru Mark Levine, M.D., chief of the Molecular and Clinical Nutrition Center at the National Institutes of Health in Washington, D.C., calls for a daily intake of about 200 milligrams.

‖ Vitamin E

When it comes to boosting immunity, vitamin E may beat out vitamin C, says Simin N. Meydani, Ph.D., chief of the nutritional immunology laboratory at the USDA Human Nutrition Research Center on Aging at Tufts University in Boston. In one study, older men and women were assigned to take 60, 200, or 800 milligrams alpha-TE (roughly the equivalent of 90, 300, or

natural WONDER

ORANGE JUICE In a study of 350 mostly healthy women, 30 percent had vitamin C levels low enough to be considered depleted. Orange juice can shore up your vitamin C stores.

1,200 IU) of vitamin E a day for 235 days, while others took a placebo. After just 4 months, those supplementing with vitamin E had a greater immune response to a variety of vaccines.

It's thought that vitamin E works to prevent the oxidation of that bad boy of the cholesterol world, low-density lipoprotein (LDL). Oxidized LDL helps cause artery walls to thicken, makes blood platelets stickier, and works in a host of ways to—bottom line—choke off blood supply to the heart. Vitamin E may also play a role in controlling diabetes.

Best food sources: Opt for vegetable and nut oils, including soybean, safflower, canola, and corn; sunflower seeds; whole grains; wheat germ; and spinach.

How much to aim for: The Daily Value for vitamin E is 30 IU—the maximum amount you'll get even from a healthy diet, including fortified breakfast cereals, says Jeffrey Blumberg, Ph.D., chief of the antioxidants research laboratory at Tufts University. Women, on average, get one-third of that, which is why it's one of the few vitamins so many experts say should be taken in supplement form.

Optimum supplementation is 100 to 400 IU for most people, 800 to 1,000 IU for those with preexisting conditions like diabetes and heart disease. If you can afford it, go for the natural version of vitamin E. It's absorbed at least 35 percent better than the synthetic form. If the bottle doesn't say "natural," look for d-alpha-tocopherol or mixed tocopherols in the ingredients list. The synthetic version is dl-alpha-tocopherol.

‖ Selenium

For decades, scientists puzzled over why residents in certain geographic areas had lower rates of some cancers. One piece of the puzzle, they now think, may be selenium.

The theories came together in a 10-year study published in the prestigious *Journal of the American Medical Association*. The researchers found that the use of a selenium supplement was associated with reduced risk of lung and colorectal (and in men, prostate) cancers by as much as two-thirds.

In test-tube studies, selenium keeps breast cancer cells from growing and induces the death of these cells. It may also play a role in suppressing angiogenesis, the growth of blood vessels that feed tumors.

Best food sources: Although the foods highest in selenium are liver, kidney, and egg yolks, you won't be eating these foods often enough to suffice if you are on a cholesterol-lowering diet. Instead, opt for seafood, whole grains, lean red meats, chicken, and mushrooms.

How much to aim for: The Daily Value for this trace mineral is 70 micrograms a day. There is no need to consider taking more than 200 micrograms a day, the amount that studies showed was effective in reducing cancer risks. (Doses above 200 micrograms must be taken under medical supervision.)

Many multivitamins don't contain selenium, so check the ingredient label carefully.

‖ Calcium

It would be so easy to get the calcium you need if you drank only milk. Yeah, and it would be so

---

Take Your Vitamins and . . . Smile

Taking a multivitamin could be one of the best ways to prevent tooth decay and gum disease. When researchers at the State University of New York at Buffalo evaluated blood samples from 9,862 men and women, they found that those with the highest vitamin A and C levels had half the rate of gum disease compared to those with the lowest levels. And high selenium levels were linked to a thirteenfold lower risk of gum disease. The reason? When the body fights bacterial invasion in dental plaque, it produces free radicals—substances looking to snatch an extra electron from other molecules in your cells—that can damage gum tissue. Antioxidant vitamins can help protect against this damage.

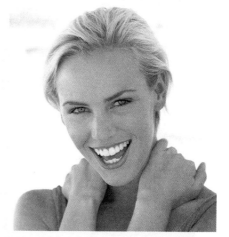

easy to quit your job and fly to Paris on the Concorde if only you won the lottery.

Reality check: Neither of these events is likely to happen.

"Women never eat or drink enough dietary sources of calcium," says Lorna Pascal, R.D., a nutrition consultant at the Dave Winfield Nutrition Center at Hackensack University Medical Center in New Jersey.

So if you are not fond of milk—and unless you're going to eat 6 ounces of tofu, plus a can of sardines with bones, 2 cups of black bean soup, and a pound of cooked spinach today and every day—you're not likely to get your recommended 1,000 to 1,500 milligrams of calcium a day from food alone. You need to take a supplement.

Best food sources: Eat dairy foods, collard greens, mustard greens, kale, canned salmon with bones, sardines with bones, corn tortillas processed with the mineral lime, tofu with calcium, and calcium-fortified citrus juice.

How much to aim for: The generic, one-size-fits-some-but-not-all Daily Value for calcium is 1,000 milligrams. Women age 51 and older need 1,500 milligrams. If you're supplementing, don't take any more than 500 milligrams at a time. The more calcium you take at one time, the less efficiently you absorb it, explains calcium expert Connie Weaver, Ph.D., professor and director of the department of foods and nutrition at Purdue University in West Lafayette, Indiana. She recommends that women divide their calcium doses throughout the day.

The tastiest source is calcium "candy"—chocolate chews containing 500 milligrams of calcium, 100 IU of vitamin D, 40 micrograms of vitamin K, and just 20 calories. Look for them wherever vitamins are sold.

‖ Vitamin D

Unless you're swigging down the cod-liver oil or relishing a meal of fatty fish like sardines or salmon three or more times a week, you have to rely mainly on the sun for your vitamin D. Today, women keep 95 percent of their bodies covered and rarely leave the sterile environs of their offices or minivans. Just how much vitamin D do you think they're making from sunlight? Not nearly enough.

If you live in a northern climate—say, anywhere north of Washington, D.C.—you're going to be hard-pressed to get sufficient vitamin D in the winter, says Michael F. Holick, M.D., Ph.D., director of the General Clinical Research Center at Boston University Medical Center. Adults who don't get enough D exacerbate their risk of osteoporosis and can develop a bone disease called osteomalacia.

Research suggests that vitamin D may also inhibit breast and colon cancers.

Best food sources: Vitamin D is found in herring, sardines, salmon, vitamin D–fortified milk, and fortified cereals, but it's difficult to get enough vitamin D from your diet, Dr. Holick says. And don't count on milk. He's done studies showing that upward of 50 percent of milk tested didn't contain even half the D touted on the label. Ten to 15 percent had none.

How much to aim for: The Daily Value for vitamin D is 400 IU, but women (and men) over age 70 should get 600 IU.

‖ Magnesium

Magnesium is easy to find in food. It's in things like dark greens, soybeans, and whole grains, foods people should eat, but often don't, says Elizabeth Somer, R.D., a nutritionist and author of *The Essential Guide to Vitamins and Minerals*. As a result, most women get around 250 milligrams of magnesium from their diets—far below the recommended Daily Value of 400 milligrams.

Magnesium plays a role in muscle contraction and in the transmission of nerve signals between cells. Your body needs magnesium to use glucose.

Some studies have shown that magnesium can reduce bone loss in postmenopausal women. One even reported an increase in bone mass in 31 women after 1 year of magnesium supplementation. But if you're postmenopausal, your body is probably getting rid of magnesium faster than you can take it in because as levels of estrogen drop, you excrete more of the mineral.

Magnesium may also reduce the risk of heart disease as well as migraine headaches and PMS.

Best food sources: Choose seafood, legumes (especially soybeans), nuts, meats, whole grains, dark green vegetables, and fat-free milk products (milk, yogurt, and cheese).

How much to aim for: The Daily Value for magnesium is 400 milligrams. Neither Tums nor multiple vitamins have enough of this vital mineral, says Somer. But don't take any more than 350 milligrams from supplements. If you have heart or kidney problems, check with your doctor before taking supplemental magnesium, and know that in some people excess magnesium may cause diarrhea.

‖ Iron

Somer knew something was wrong when she was pregnant with her second child. She was exhausted, but when she complained to her doctor, he reassured her that her anemia test was negative, figuratively patted her on the head, and blamed it on the pregnancy.

As a nutritionist, however, Somer knew better. She went for a serum ferritin test—a more sensitive blood test that measures iron deficiency before it becomes anemia. A normal score is 20; hers was 4.

Hence her philosophy: "I recommend that every woman of childbearing age have a serum ferritin test done. And be feisty about it. Find out what your value is. Because every single woman that has come to me complaining of tiredness who had the test done was iron deficient."

Overall, studies show that between 30 and 80 percent of women are iron deficient. Not anemic, just low. The symptoms are similar, says Somer: fatigue, breathlessness from walking up a flight of stairs, increased susceptibility to colds and infections, and muddled thinking.

Best food sources: You can get iron from red meats, poultry, eggs, legumes, Cream of Wheat cereal, baked potatoes, soybeans, pumpkin seeds, and clams.

How much to aim for: The Daily Value for iron is 18 milligrams. Women who menstruate heavily or use an IUD should get more, up to 25 milligrams, says Somer.

‖ B Vitamins

A family of B vitamins—B_6, B_{12}, folate, thiamin, riboflavin, niacin, pantothenic acid, and biotin—are particularly important to women for a variety of reasons, not the least of which is that they help their bodies break down food for energy. Without them, you'd be even more exhausted.

The three B vitamins women need most are folate (also known as folic acid) and vitamins B_6 and B_{12}. Together, they control levels of homocysteine, an amino acid that has been linked to an increased risk of heart disease and stroke. At least one major study, the Nurses' Health Study, shows that women who consume high amounts of folate and vitamin B_6, from either food or supplements, have a risk of developing heart disease that's nearly half that of women who get lower amounts.

Best food sources: Foods high in folate include fortified cereals, beans, asparagus, spinach, broccoli, and brussels sprouts. To get more vitamin B_6, go for leafy greens, potatoes, bananas, avocados, chicken, beef, fish, brown rice, and peanuts. Vitamin B_{12} is available from meat, seafood, and dairy products. Breakfast cereals and soy products are often fortified with it.

How much to aim for: The Daily Value for folate for nonpregnant women is 400 micrograms a day. For vitamin B_6, the Daily Value is 2 milligrams. John M. Ellis, M.D., author of *Vitamin B_6 Therapy*, recommends between 50 to 100 milligrams for most adults. Don't take more than 100 milligrams of B_6 a day without your doctor's supervision. At high doses, vitamin B_6 can cause nerve damage.

For vitamin B_{12}, the Daily Value is 6 micrograms. If you're 50 or older, chances are that you may have trouble absorbing it from food. So the Institute of Medicine at the National Academy of Sciences says that people 50 and older should get their B_{12} in crystalline form. A multivitamin should more than meet your needs. Some researchers have raised the bar on B_{12} and now recommend 25 micrograms, and some manufacturers are adding this amount to their "senior" supplements.

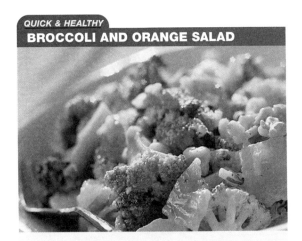

QUICK & HEALTHY
BROCCOLI AND ORANGE SALAD

Broccoli and oranges team up for a double dose of flavor and lots of antioxidants (like vitamin C) and the B vitamin folate. Turn ordinary meals into something special with this unique alternative to dressed lettuce.

4	cups bite-size broccoli florets
¼	cup orange juice
1	tablespoon white balsamic or white wine vinegar
1	tablespoon soy sauce
1	tablespoon olive oil
½	teaspoon Dijon mustard
2	large oranges, peeled and sectioned
⅓	cup finely chopped red onion

Steam the broccoli until crisp-tender.

In a large bowl, whisk together the orange juice, vinegar, soy sauce, oil, and mustard. Add the oranges and onion. Toss gently. Add the broccoli and toss gently to combine. Serve at room temperature or chilled.

MAKES 4 SERVINGS

Per serving: 100 calories, 4 g protein, 16 g carbohydrates, 4 g fat, 0 mg cholesterol, 4 g dietary fiber, 291 mg sodium

CHAPTER 6

Are Your Hormones Making You Fat?

Get a handle on hormone-related cravings with this new approach to emotional eating.

K aren led a typical time-pressed life: She had two young children at home and a husband who'd sold his business, retired early, and was always underfoot. Even though they could afford it, her husband refused to hire any household help, so Karen's days were a blur of child care, meal preparation, and housekeeping.

In between, she ate. Cake and ice cream at children's birthday parties. Chips and snacks bought for the kids. Leftover dessert and mashed potatoes from dinner. It didn't take long for Karen's weight to creep up, prompting her to seek help from a weight-loss clinic.

"Why do you eat these things?" asked the nutritionist Karen consulted.

"Because I like to eat," she said.

"Why do you eat these things?" the nutritionist repeated.

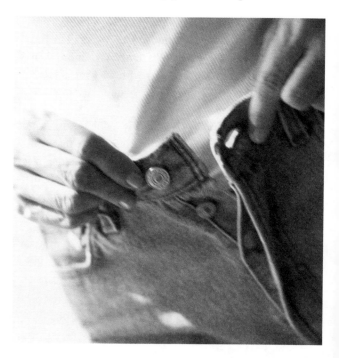

"Because it tastes good."

The nutritionist just looked at her, waiting for the real answer.

"Because it makes me feel good," Karen finally admitted.

As a child, Karen only had time to herself when she ate. If she was reading or playing, for example, her mother piled on more chores. But mealtime was sacrosanct. So Karen learned that eating equals time for herself, says Judith J. Wurtman, Ph.D., a research scientist in the department of brain and cognitive sciences at MIT in Cambridge, Massachusetts, who worked with Karen.

"If you had one wish, what would you wish for?" Dr. Wurtman asked Karen.

"An hour a day to myself," came the answer.

So Dr. Wurtman convinced Karen's husband to hire a babysitter to watch the kids for at least 2 hours a day so that his wife had time alone. Voilà! With Karen's needs met in ways other than eating, her mindless eating stopped, and she started to drop the extra pounds.

Be Your Own Food Therapist

If you're like most women, you can identify with Karen in some way. The bucket of leftover fried chicken devoured one rainy Saturday while trapped indoors with the kids. The doughnuts consumed after a frustrating meeting at the office. The oversize bag of potato chips that disappeared after the stressful phone call to your mother.

No one disputes the connection between food and mood, says Mindy Kurzer, Ph.D., associate professor of food science and nutrition at the University of Minnesota in St. Paul. "Food crav-

ings are not 'all in your head,' and they're not trivial."

What is less clear is the cause. You eat for lots of reasons, ranging from hunger to boredom to the social settings in which you find yourself. But in recent years, researchers have zeroed in on another reason: the complex network of neurotransmitters and other chemicals in our bodies that turn our appetites on and off. When these various chemicals get out of whack, so can your eating habits.

Elizabeth Somer, R.D., calls it the cascade of chemicals. All day long, you're "riding the swells of chemical surges," says Somer, a nutritionist and author of *Food and Mood*. There are 20 to 30 different hormones, neurotransmitters, enzymes, and amino acids in your body that contribute to your eating habits, including the following:

Galanin. A neuropeptide, galanin stimulates your desire for fats and carbohydrates.

Neuropeptide Y. This neurotransmitter triggers carbohydrate cravings.

Endorphins. These are the same chemicals that give you a supercharged feeling after running 3 miles. Eating something sweet like chocolate produces the same feeling.

Serotonin. Of all the chemical messengers that have been studied, serotonin has received the greatest attention, primarily for its ability to improve sleep, diminish pain, and reduce appetite.

The Menstrual Mood Cycle

It's like clockwork. Ten days before your period, you're craving things like chocolate, macaroni and cheese, and baked potatoes. Anything sweet, starchy, or creamy—and plentiful.

Why Women Crave Chocolate

It's the ultimate indulgence. No other food is craved the way chocolate is, especially by women. Researchers don't know why, but some think it's because chocolate is mainly made up of sugar and fat. The combination seems to send those feel-good brain chemicals, known as endorphins, into the stratosphere.

Adding to chocolate's appeal is its unique melt-in-your-mouth texture, says Clara E. Gerhardt, Ph.D., associate professor of human development and family studies at Samford University in Birmingham, Alabama, who specializes in food issues.

You can give in to chocolate with some guilt-free alternatives suggested by Elizabeth Somer, R.D., a nutritionist and author of *Food and Mood*.

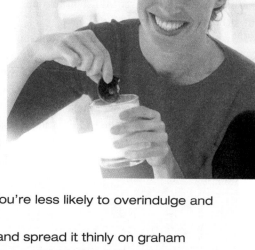

- Instead of using hard chocolate in baking, try cocoa powder, which has fewer calories.
- Dip pieces of fruit into low-fat chocolate syrup.
- Eat chocolate with meals, not as a snack. You're less likely to overindulge and more likely to choose a small portion.
- Warm reduced-fat fudge in the microwave and spread it thinly on graham crackers for a snack that's low in fat.

It's not in your mind. It's in your hormones.

Women eat more between the time they ovulate and the time their periods start. One theory blames it on increased levels of the female hormone progesterone. You know how this works if you've ever tracked your temperature while trying to get pregnant and seen it rise ½ degree just after ovulation. A higher body temperature burns more calories, impelling you to reach for more food.

Studies show that the dip in estrogen just before your period reduces serotonin and endorphins, making you hungrier. And lowered endorphins make you reach for the sweet stuff. That's right: c-h-o-c-o-l-a-t-e.

These cravings are not much different from what you typically experience during the month; they just get stronger and more intense before your periods, says Louise Dye, Ph.D., associate professor of psychology at the University of Leeds in England.

What to do? Give in. To bump up the serotonin, eat what Somer calls anti-PMS foods.

For breakfast: Try whole grain cereal sprinkled with wheat germ in fat-free milk, a piece of whole wheat toast spread with all-fruit jam, and grapefruit juice.

For lunch: Fix yourself a chicken breast sandwich with sprouts and honey mustard on whole wheat bread, carrot-raisin-apple salad, melon balls, fat-free milk, and ice water with lemon.

For dinner: Stir-fry tofu and vegetables with safflower oil, and have them with brown rice and 1% milk.

In the midmorning and midafternoon: Snack on either a whole wheat tortilla with 1 tablespoon of low-fat peanut butter or half a whole wheat bagel with fat-free cream cheese and carrot juice.

But if it's the cravings talking and only sweet, creamy foods will do, then have them—in moderation. Start with a small piece of chocolate or a couple of Hershey's Kisses, for example. Then you'll avoid what Dr. Dye calls the what-the-hell effect, as in, "I ate one bite, I may as well eat it all."

The Land of Comfort Food

It may be Mallomars or mashed potatoes, macaroni and cheese or even something weird like a can of sweetened condensed milk. We all have our food anchors, stemming from associations between what we see, hear, taste, smell, or touch, and from various experiences, says Karen Miller-Kovach, R.D., lead scientist for Weight Watchers International in Woodbury, New York.

No Bad Foods

When did eating certain foods become immoral? As in, "I'll be good and order the salad instead of the fries." Or, "I was so bad last night. I ate two brownies."

Food is food. Eating it or not eating it doesn't make you a good or bad person.

Yet at least one study has shown what we all know: Chocolate addicts feel guilty when they eat their favorite food, leading the scientists to conclude that no matter how much pleasure a food provides, if you think you're eating too much, then any pleasure will be short-lived, accompanied by feelings of guilt.

"Why a woman can sit down and eat fat-free frozen yogurt and feel like it's a good food, but if she eats premium Häagen-Dazs, it's a bad food, I'll never understand," says Karen Miller-Kovach, R.D., lead scientist for Weight Watchers International in Woodbury, New York.

The only way to change this thinking, says Miller-Kovach, is to challenge your internal beliefs. Do you really believe that Ben and Jerry's will kill you and sorbet will make you live to be 100? Probably not.

Think about it: Three cups of low-fat yogurt has the same amount of fat as ½ cup of premium ice cream. So there's absolutely nothing wrong with eating what you really want. And in fact, if it's more satisfying, it's the "right" thing to do.

"If, when you were a little kid and scraped your knee, your mother gave you a chocolate chip cookie to help pacify you, that routine established a connection between the chocolate chip cookie—the anchor—and feeling better," says Miller-Kovach. Then when you're 40 and your teenage son yells that he hates you, you automatically reach for the cookie jar.

The key is to become aware. Even though many women find it a bother, Miller-Kovach stands by the tried-and-true food diary.

• For 1 week, write down everything you put in your mouth. Then record what you're feeling, where you are, and what you're thinking and doing. Do it just after you swallow—or you'll forget.

• Read your diary carefully, noting the patterns. It's important to do this after the week is over so that you can detect patterns that are not usually apparent in the heat of the eating moment, Dr. Kurzer explains.

"The key questions to ask are, 'Why was I overeating? What did it get for me?'" says Miller-Kovach.

To detour around comfort food land mines:

• Find nonfood things that you can do to fill that same need. If it's indulgence you're after, take a bubble bath or a nap, or curl up with a stack of glossy magazines.

• Understand the feeling. Keeping a journal or doing some creative writing can be a wonderful way of understanding the emotion that sends you running for the Häagen-Dazs.

• Have ready a list of at least five alternatives to the food. If you have only one and you can't do it at that time, you'll just give up and eat.

The idea is to create new anchors. It's kind of like biofeedback, only you don't need a fancy machine.

Say you feel tense every morning when you enter the office, so you make a beeline for the doughnuts. Instead, think about a time when you felt relaxed. For one woman, it was when she rocked her son. She trained herself to connect twirling her wedding ring with that memory and learned to twirl her ring whenever she entered her office.

CHAPTER 7

The Women's Health Companion

Protect yourself against seven women-only problems with foods, herbs, and supplements.

As the saying goes, if men menstruated, women would be allowed to take sick days during their periods. But men don't, so women are left to find ways to deal with PMS, breast discomfort, and other problems that plague their unique anatomy.

Fortunately, help isn't hard to find. Most women-only health conditions can be treated and prevented with foods, herbs, and supplements. These natural remedies enable you to take charge of your health. By learning how to use natural remedies, you can find the power to replenish, rejuvenate, and refresh yourself.

But natural remedies are no substitute for your doctor and conventional medicine. Always consult with your doctor before taking herbs and supplements. And tell your doctor about any chronic symptoms you may have.

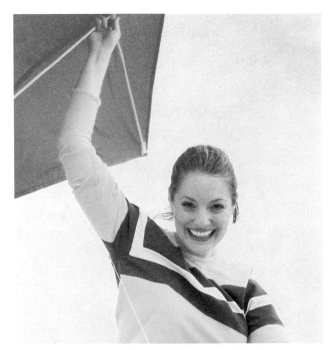

‖ Breast Discomfort

The next time your breasts feel sore and tender, you may want to blame your period. Right before and during menstruation, higher-than-usual levels of the female hormone estrogen may cause one or both breasts to swell and become sensitive. Assuming that your doctor has assured you that you have nothing serious to worry about, your best bet for relief may be one of these remedies.

Eat less fat. Women in cultures that consume a low-fat diet have fewer breast complaints than women who eat high-fat diets. Ellen Yankauskas, M.D., director of the Women's Center for Family Health in Atascadero, California, advises those who experience breast discomfort to eat a diet consisting of less than 30 percent fat. (On an 1,800-calories-per-day diet, that's no more than 60 grams of fat.)

Try some vitamin E. "There are some studies that have shown taking slightly larger amounts of vitamin E to be very effective in relieving breast tenderness and discomfort," says Dr. Yankauskas. Take 200 to 400 IU of vitamin E a day.

‖ Fibrocystic Breast Changes

A condition affecting half of all women at some point in their lives, fibrocystic breast changes occur when fluid-filled sacs form in the breast's milk-producing glands. You can relax; this condition does not increase your risk of breast cancer. Still, the pain and lumpiness, which often intensify before menstruation, can be frustrating and uncomfortable.

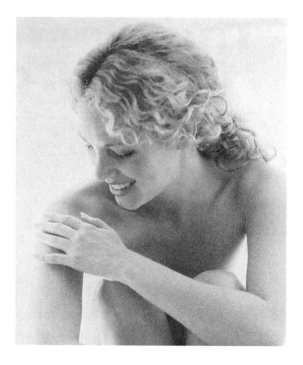

While experts aren't sure what brings about these breast changes, some suspect higher-than-normal amounts of estrogen and prolactin, the milk-release hormone. To reduce your chances of developing fibrocystic breasts, these dietary strategies can help.

Be prudent about fat. Some evidence suggests that women who consume a lot of dietary fat—especially the saturated fat in butter, bacon, and other animal foods—are more likely to develop fibrocystic breast changes. This is probably because a high-fat diet increases the amount of estrogen circulating in a woman's body, which can fuel the growth of breast lumps. In one small study, 10 women with fibrocystic breasts reduced their intake of dietary fat to 20 percent of their total daily calories. Three months later, all of them said that their pain was gone.

Cut the coffee. Researchers at Yale University School of Medicine found that women who drink about two cups of coffee a day (containing from 31 to 250 milligrams of caffeine) were 150 percent more likely to develop fibrocystic changes than women getting no caffeine. That may be due to coffee's content of methylxanthines, compounds that can cause breast lumps to become inflamed and tender. In a study at Ohio State University in Columbus, 45 women who drank an average of four cups of coffee a day quit cold turkey. After 2 months, 37 of the women—82 percent—said that their breast lumps were gone.

‖ Fibroids

An estimated 20 to 40 percent of all women have fibroids—noncancerous tumors that grow on the inside or outside lining of the uterus, or within its muscular wall. These growths can be as small as a pea or as large as a grapefruit. While experts aren't exactly sure what causes fibroids, they do know that they occur most often when a woman's estrogen levels are high—when she's pregnant, for example, or if she's taking the Pill.

Not all fibroids cause symptoms or need treatment. But some women experience a variety of bothersome or uncomfortable symptoms, including heavy bleeding, pressure in the abdomen, abdominal or lower-back pain, and frequent urination. If you want to avoid these symptoms, consider this advice.

Go vegetarian. Preliminary evidence suggests that fibroids are linked to a meat-heavy diet and that eating lots of green veggies seems to be protective. Researchers in Italy compared 843 women with fibroids to 1,557 women without. Those with fibroids reported eating significantly more red meat and fewer servings of green vegetables. It's known that a diet high in meat raises a woman's levels of estrogen, which seems to increase the risk of developing fibroids. Premenopausal vegetarian women have blood estrogen levels that are 15 to 20 percent lower than those of their meat-eating sisters.

‖ Menopause

You already knew that menopause could affect your mood, sex drive, and memory, as well as your heart and bones. But here's another, less-discussed menopausal change: digestive symptoms, from indigestion and heartburn to bloating, gas, constipation, and even gallstones. Fortunately, all of these symptoms will disappear with the right adjustments in your eating habits.

Enjoy frequent, small meals. Try five or six mini-meals instead of the traditional big three, suggests Larrian Gillespie, M.D., author of *The Menopause Diet*. Dr. Gillespie recommends eating no more than 250 to 300 calories per meal.

Focus on fruits, vegetables, and whole grains. To avoid bloating, gas, and constipation, Dr. Gillespie recommends choosing high-fiber goodies such as fruits and vegetables.

Indulge in a bit of butter. Eating a small amount of dietary fat in one sitting—10 grams per day—can stimulate the gallbladder to empty, preventing the formation of gallstones. "Melt a scant tablespoon of unsalted butter, and use it to dip your veggies," says Dr. Gillespie. (If you already have gallstones, don't try this.) But keep total fat intake to about 40 grams a day.

Premenstrual Syndrome

Perhaps the only nice thing to say about a problem that plagues 30 to 40 percent of women with bloating, achy breasts, depression, restlessness, and weepiness is this: A poll found that 79 percent of men surveyed felt that women are not malingering—PMS is a bona fide health condition.

And there is convincing evidence that what you eat (or don't eat) during this touchy 7 to 14 days can make a significant difference in how you feel, both physically and emotionally. The following strategies may spare you from PMS symptoms.

Drink more milk. Getting more calcium into your diet may help ease premenstrual moodiness and discomfort. Researchers had 466 women with documented PMS take either 1,200 milligrams of calcium (in supplement form) or placebos. By the second menstrual cycle, the pain, foul moods, food cravings, and bloating of the women taking calcium began to improve. By their third cycle, their symptoms were reduced by 48 percent, compared with 30 percent in the placebo group. It's possible to get this amount of calcium through food. One cup of calcium-enriched orange juice contains 300 milligrams of calcium, the same amount as in 1 cup of milk and 25 percent of the amount used in the study for premenopausal symptoms.

Allow chocolate its place. A scientific review of the sweet and creamy delight suggests that chocolate cravings kick into high gear

Go Vegan to Curb Cramps

A low-fat vegetarian diet gave relief to 33 women with moderate to severe menstrual cramps and PMS, according to new research from Georgetown University in Washington, D.C. Pain duration and intensity were significantly reduced—and so were PMS symptoms. The women shunned meat, fish, dairy, and eggs, as well as butter, oils, and even peanut butter, says lead study author Neal Barnard, M.D., president of the Physicians' Committee for Responsible Medicine in Washington, D.C.

The diet derives about 10 percent of calories from fat—the lowest healthy limit. The good news: Results come quickly. Following the plan for just one or two menstrual cycles should be enough to help you determine if it's going to work for you. "After a month or two, if you want to try adding back other foods, go ahead," says Dr. Barnard.

before a woman's period and may be related to, among other things, fluctuating hormone levels. So if you crave chocolate, indulge—in moderation.

Cut back on fat. The kind of fat you eat before your period—and how much of it you eat—can affect the severity of your symptoms. The worst kind of fat, not surprisingly, is the saturated kind found in meats, whole-fat dairy foods, and many processed foods. Saturated fat causes estrogen levels to rise, which worsens virtually all PMS symptoms. All women, not just those with PMS, are advised to limit their consumption of fat to no more than 25 percent of total calories, with 7 percent coming from saturated fat and the rest from unsaturated fat.

Feast on fish. Preliminary evidence suggests that having too few omega-3s and too much linolenic acid (an unsaturated fat) in your system can lead to an overproduction of a certain type of prostaglandin. This hormonelike compound can cause menstrual cramps. Omega-3 fatty acids can be found in canola and flaxseed oils and fatty fish.

Urinary Tract Infections

Each year, an estimated 26 million women endure the frustrating symptoms of urinary tract infections (UTIs). Usually caused when bacteria take up residence in the urethra (the tube through which urine flows), the symptoms of a

natural
WONDER
CHASTEBERRY
The herb chasteberry may be a powerful ally in your war against PMS. It limits the production of the hormone prolactin, thus relieving PMS symptoms.

UTI include an urgent need to urinate and pain or burning upon urination. Women are 25 times more likely to get UTIs than men because their urethras are shorter, making it easier for bacteria to migrate there from the nearby rectal area. Want to let these bugs know they're not welcome? Fight back with these remedies.

Sip some cranberry juice. Cranberry juice has long been a home remedy for urinary tract infections, and for good reason. In one study, researchers in Boston gave 153 older women 10 ounces of sweetened cranberry juice a day. After 6 months, the cranberry juice drinkers were 42 percent less likely to have urinary tract bacteria in their urine than women who drank a look-alike juice. To prevent bladder infections, drink 10 ounces of cranberry juice a

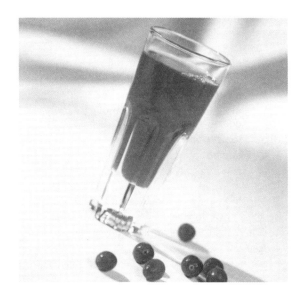

day. (Because cranberry juice packs a lot of calories, you may want to opt for artificially sweetened cranberry juice.)

Nibble on blueberries. Like cranberries, they contain condensed tannins, compounds that also give bladder walls a Teflon-like coating. Research suggests that it takes about 1 cup of blueberries a day, fresh or frozen, to prevent recurrent UTIs.

Enjoy a cup of yogurt. Yogurt contains *Lactobacillus acidophilus*, which may create an acidic environment and prevent the growth of unwanted bacteria. The scientific evidence is still somewhat controversial, however, regarding just how effective it is for preventing infections. Some

experts recommend that you eat a cup of yogurt made with active live cultures daily.

‖ Yeast Infections

Yeast infection is the second most common vaginal infection in North America. It's an itchy, miserable affliction that finds 45 percent of women more than once. Most often, yeast infections are caused by the organism *Candida albicans*.

Normally, candida, which lives mostly in the intestines and the vagina, coexists peacefully with other microorganisms. But any number of factors

---

QUICK & HEALTHY

CRANBERRY RELISH WITH APPLES AND CURRANTS

The plentiful cranberries in this tart-sweet sauce contain condensed tannins, which help to combat urinary tract infections. This version has apples, sweet currants, and walnuts added to the mix.

¾	cup + 1 tablespoon sugar
1	cup hot water
1	bag (12 ounces) cranberries
1	medium Granny Smith apple, peeled, cored, and chopped
2½	tablespoons currants
⅛	teaspoon ground cloves
¼	cup coarsely chopped walnuts

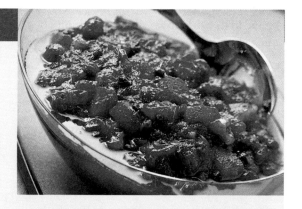

Stir the sugar into the water in a medium saucepan over low heat. Simmer the mixture for 2 to 3 minutes to dissolve the sugar, stirring once or twice.

Stir in the cranberries and apple and simmer, uncovered, for 8 to 10 minutes, or until the berries have popped and the sauce has thickened. Stir in the currants and cloves and let the sauce cool. Stir in the nuts.

MAKES 10 SERVINGS (ABOUT 3 CUPS)
Per serving: 136 calories, 1 g protein, 30 g carbohydrates, 2 g fat, 0 mg cholesterol, 1 g dietary fiber, 1 mg sodium

There's Such a Thing as "Too Clean"

If you douche, use a vinegar-and-water solution (2 tablespoons of white vinegar per 1 quart of water). And don't douche more than once a week—it will kill off "good" bacteria.

can destroy the so-called friendly bacteria in the vagina that normally keep yeast in check, causing candida to grow out of control. These include antibiotics, poor diet, and pregnancy.

You can regain the upper hand on candida with help from these dietary changes.

Feast on ½ cup of yogurt daily. Most women have heard that yogurt—specifically, the live bacteria in yogurt called *Lactobacillus acidophilus*—is a potent home remedy for yeast infections. In addition, research suggests that it

works for another common type of vaginal infection, called bacterial vaginitis.

Flavor your food with garlic. Garlic contains a crew of chemical compounds, among them ajoene, allicin/alliin, and diallyl sulfide, all proven to fight fungal infections. In one animal study, mice with yeast infections were given either a solution made with aged garlic extract or an inactive saline solution. Two days later, the rats given saline were still infected. But those in the garlic group were completely fungus-free.

Breast Cancer Alert

Your best defense against this killer: Combine cutting-edge dietary strategies with conventional medicine.

As soon as you find the lump in your breast, you feel the terror welling up inside you. And when, after the breast exam, mammogram, and biopsy, you're told you have cancer, suddenly conventional medicine just doesn't seem as comforting as it did before.

To be sure, you should not ignore your doctor's advice to have chemotherapy, surgery, radiation treatments, or other conventional methods of therapy. But you can dramatically increase your chances of beating the disease and lower your risk of recurrence with *Prevention*'s revolutionary food plan.

Plenty of doctors will tell you, "We simply need more research before we know if food remedies really work against cancer." But once you have that diagnosis in hand, do you really want to wait for all of that research to come in?

That's why *Prevention* designed the Eat to Beat Breast Cancer Diet. Based on groundbreaking research, this ultrahealthy eating plan will not only help you wage your battle against cancer but also increase your energy, helping you to withstand the rigors of chemotherapy.

The Eat to Beat Breast Cancer Diet

For the Eat to Beat Breast Cancer Diet, you'll meander a bit from the government's Food Guide Pyramid. Here's what you'll be eating.

Three to six servings of whole grain foods a day. Throw away your white rice, white bread, and white pasta and switch to whole grain foods made from barley, quinoa,

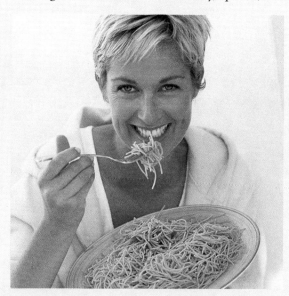

spelt, oats, bulgur, wheatberries, and whole wheat. This simple switch will maximize your fiber intake, in turn lowering levels of estrogen in your body. It's high levels of estrogen that have been linked with breast cancer.

To find foods made from whole grains, become a label detective. Make sure *whole* wheat, oats, or another grain is one of the first ingredients listed. Once you know what to look for on the label, track your intake of whole wheat bread, pasta, cereal, rice, and other whole grain products.

One to two servings of beans a day. As with whole grains, beans supply a great fiber boost. Eventually, your gastrointestinal tract will adapt, but if you find that beans make you gassy, add a few drops of Beano or another natural enzyme product.

To get more beans into your diet, try these tips.
• Sample bean-rich goodies such as falafel (chickpea balls), hummus (chickpea dip), or black bean burritos.
• Toss drained, canned chickpeas into a salad.
• Include canned beans in soups, stews, even pasta.

A handful of nuts several times a week. Nuts are a great source of fiber and monounsaturated fats—another likely breast cancer foe. You can eat them straight from the package or try mixing them in your whole grain oatmeal for a two-in-one anti-breast-cancer punch. When buying nuts, look for raw, unsalted types. Avoid nuts that come with a coating, which could add unnecessary and possibly problematic hydrogenated fats.

Nine or more servings of fruits and vegetables a day. Of all the ele-

Vegetable Power

To sneak more vegetables into your daily fare, try the following:

• Use convenience veggies, which are just as healthy overall as whole fresh produce. That includes frozen, canned, salad bar, and precut.
• Count 100 percent juice for two of your daily servings but concentrate on the most nutrient-packed varieties: citrus, Concord grape, carrot, tomato, and vegetable juice cocktail.
• Make a shopping list, then be prepared for a shock: Your grocery cart will look like it's swimming with veggies at first. But if you stick with this plan, you'll soon be surprised by the lack of veggies in other people's carts.

ments of the Eat to Beat Breast Cancer Diet, this one is probably the most important. Fruits and vegetables are packed with promising cancer-fighting phytochemicals that help create a biochemical environment that maximizes your ability to resist cancer.

Getting nine servings a day, however, takes thought and planning. Aim for three servings at each meal plus fruit or veggie snacks each day. Every single day, try to include something from each of these groups.
• Cruciferous veggies: broccoli, broccoli sprouts, brussels sprouts, cabbage, cauliflower
• Lycopene-rich produce: tomatoes, red grapefruit, watermelon, guava

- Beta-carotene-rich produce: winter squash, carrots, sweet potatoes
- Citrus fruits: oranges, grapefruit
- Berries: strawberries, raspberries, blueberries, blackberries
- Dark green leafy veggies: spinach, romaine, kale, collards, Swiss chard

If you don't exactly love vegetables, judiciously use cheese, oils, and nuts to make veggies taste seductively rich, the way the French do. A major bonus: Adding some fat to your veggies means that you'll absorb tons more of the carotenoids—crucial cancer fighters, such as the beta-carotene found in carrots—which are fat soluble.

Shiitake mushrooms and artichokes once a week. These gems are powerful cancer fighters because of an ingredient that they have in common: silymarin. Also found in the herb milk thistle, silymarin supports optimal liver function.

One to two servings of low-fat dairy products a day. Dairy fat has a high concentration of a molecule called conjugated linoleic acid (CLA), which has promising anti-cancer activity. So you're actually better off with 1% milk rather than fat-free.

Try to find an organic, non-BST milk, however. (BST is a growth hormone.) Milk from non-BST cows contains lesser amounts of a compound called IGF-1. Higher blood levels of IGF-1 have been linked with several types of cancer.

One to two servings of soy products a day. Soybeans contain many potentially anticarcinogenic compounds, including saponins, phytates, protease inhibitors, and isoflavones (weak estrogen compounds). In Japan, where women eat much more soy than we do in the States, the incidence of breast cancer is much lower.

You can get soy in many forms, including tofu, soy burgers, soy dogs, soy milk, soy cheese, soy sausage, miso, soy nuts, and so on. Experiment with different brands; you'll find that you like some brands better than others.

Soy for Breast Cancer: Good or Bad?

Confusion and controversy surround the inclusion of soy in the diets of those women with estrogen-positive, postmenopausal breast cancer who are being treated with the drug tamoxifen. Do the weak phytoestrogens in soy fuel cancer growth, are they neutral, or are they possibly beneficial for reducing cancer risk? Do they compete with tamoxifen and make it less effective, or do they actually enhance its benefits?

Though a few cancer specialists advise women in this category to avoid soy foods because of the weak estrogen compounds they contain, many believe that one or two servings a day of whole soy foods (such as those that the Japanese consume) will not be harmful. Just stay away from soy powders or soy pills that contain isolated isoflavones.

QUICK & HEALTHY
PHYTOCHEMICAL SUPER SHAKE

This shake gives you one serving of vegetables, two servings of fruit, one serving of soy, one serving of ground flaxseed, and one serving of whole grain (wheat bran plus wheat germ)—plus one-third of your daily fiber. It's also delicious!

2½	**ounces soft or silken tofu (about ⅓ cup)**
6	**baby carrots**
¾	**cup fresh or frozen unsweetened fruit**
1	**tablespoon wheat bran**
1	**tablespoon wheat germ**
1	**tablespoon ground flaxseed**
¾	**cup calcium-fortified soy milk**
¾	**cup calcium-fortified orange juice**

In a blender, combine the tofu, carrots, fruit, wheat bran, wheat germ, flaxseed, soy milk, and orange juice. Process on low speed, then increase to high for 1 to 3 minutes, or until fully blended.

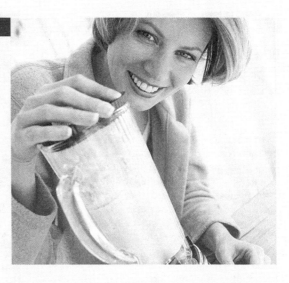

MAKES 3 CUPS

Per shake: 313 calories, 18 g protein, 49 g carbohydrates, 9 g fat, 9 g dietary fiber, 565 mg calcium, 89 mg sodium

Fatty fish two or three times a week. The omega-3 fats in fish such as salmon, mackerel, white tuna, sardines, and herring may help fight breast cancer.

Try to make fish your main protein source. That will help you cut back on meat and poultry, significantly lowering your intake of saturated fats. If you don't want to cut back on meat, buy only very lean cuts and keep your portions small (the size of a deck of playing cards or less).

Garlic, herbs, and spices as often as you wish. Garlic kills breast cancer cells in the test tube—and maybe in you. But if you cook garlic, always peel and chop, then let it rest for 10 to 15 minutes before you heat it so that the cancer-fighting compounds have time to develop.

Besides garlic, every herb or spice that you add to your meals increases your intake of phytochemicals that may fight cancer.

One to 2 tablespoons of ground flaxseed a day. Flax is a source of lignan precursors, which are converted inside the body to a weak antiestrogen that may be useful in preventing or treating estrogen-responsive tumors. Flax also supplies a plant form of omega-3 fats.

For your body to digest flax, the seeds must be ground. You can grind them yourself in a coffee grinder or simply buy flax meal, which has been ground for you.

Four to six cups of green tea, either hot or iced, a day. Both black

I DID IT!

Nancy Brinker:
How One Breast Cancer Survivor Fought Back

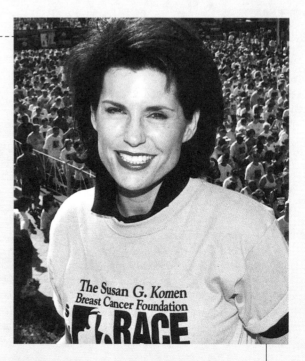

Breast cancer made a big mistake when it claimed Nancy Brinker's sister, Susan Komen, at the tender age of 36. Like Bruce Wayne vowing to avenge his murdered parents, Brinker swore to go after the dreaded disease as if it were a street thug.

She created the Susan G. Komen Breast Cancer Foundation in Dallas and went to work battling the disease. Today, nearly 20 years later, the foundation has raised more than $200 million, making it the world's largest private funder of breast cancer research.

Ironically, one of the first lives saved by the foundation was Nancy's own.

It was at one of their very first events— a breast health fair in Dallas—that she discovered her own cancer. "In 1984, at this early educational event that we sponsored, I absentmindedly ran my hand across a breast 'form' (a soft, realistic model) that was there to teach women what a cancer might feel like and felt the lump inside," she says. Later that night, she noticed a lump in her breast that felt the same way. It turned out to be cancer.

Brinker had a modified radical mastectomy in which her breast was removed. The cancer was the same kind that had killed her sister, so many lymph nodes were also removed. Five months of chemotherapy followed, along with a wide range of complementary therapies.

"I took a lot of vitamins during my chemo. I prayed, and prayed, and prayed," she says. "And I did a lot of visualization: I would fill myself with bright white light and visualize it going after any cancer cells. During my rehab, I was in support groups that included lots of children, and I learned how important laughter is. It's a great stress buster and mood changer."

Intensive yearly checkups show that, more than 15 years later, Brinker is still cancer-free. "I still take lots of vitamins, particularly antioxidants. I also use herbs to help boost my immune system and relieve the stress caused by my hectic schedule. I walk 4 to 5 miles every day, follow a Mediterranean-style diet, and try to incorporate some humor—something to help me laugh— into every day."

To learn more about the Susan G. Komen Breast Cancer Foundation and the Komen Race for the Cure series, call (800) I'M AWARE (462-9273).

KALE-POTATO-TOMATO BAKE

Here's a luscious way to get more cancer-fighting kale into your diet.

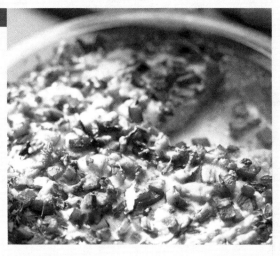

2	tablespoons olive oil
1	large onion, finely chopped
3	medium potatoes, peeled and cut into ¼" cubes
1	box (10 ounces) frozen chopped kale, thawed and well-drained
1	can (14½ ounces) diced tomatoes, drained
1	container (15 ounces) reduced-fat ricotta cheese
½	cup shredded reduced-fat Monterey Jack cheese
2	eggs, lightly beaten, or ½ cup fat-free liquid egg substitute
½	teaspoon salt

Preheat oven to 350°F. Coat a 13" × 9" baking dish with cooking spray.

In a large nonstick skillet, warm the oil over medium heat. Add the onion and cook, stirring often, for 3 minutes. Add the potatoes and cook, stirring occasionally, for 15 minutes, or until tender. Add the kale and tomatoes. Cook for 1 minute.

In a large bowl, whisk together the ricotta, Monterey Jack, eggs, and salt. Add the kale mixture and stir to combine. Spoon into the baking dish.

Bake for 40 minutes, or until a knife inserted in the center comes out clean. Let stand on a wire rack for 10 minutes before serving.

MAKES 6 SERVINGS

Per serving: 284 calories, 17 g protein, 24 g carbohydrates, 14 g fat, 99 mg cholesterol, 3 g dietary fiber, 710 mg sodium

and green teas contain flavonoids, compounds that possess protective antioxidant properties. The flavonoids in both types of tea keep dangerous LDL cholesterol in check, reducing the plaque that can clog arteries. But green tea seems to be a more potent anticancer weapon than black. Both green and black teas come from the same plant, but they are processed differently. Unlike black tea, green contains an anticancer compound known as epigallocatechin gallate (EGCG).

Extra-virgin olive oil or canola oil for cooking. Both of these oils are high in monounsaturated fats, which may protect against breast cancer. Besides using these oils in your cooking and salad dressings, buy processed foods with no trans fats (from partially hydrogenated oils), because trans fats may increase cancer risk.

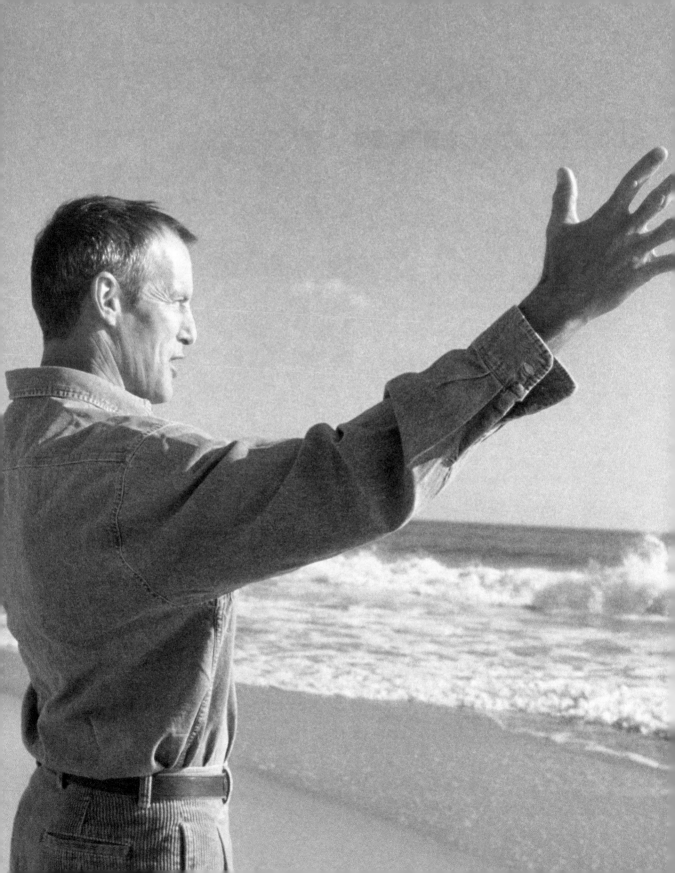

PART FOUR

For Men Only

Fight disease—and enhance your sex life—with natural remedies just for men.

CHAPTER 8

Save a Life—Yours

These symptoms should make you think twice about canceling that doctor's appointment.

During the 1970 NBA Finals, New York Knicks center Willis Reed sustained a painful thigh injury that should have sidelined him for the rest of the series. But Reed limped onto the court for the deciding game and, to cheers from the hometown crowd, scored the first two points, then went on to lead his team to the championship.

In the minds of many men, Reed became a legend for upholding that peculiarly male commandment: Thou shalt not acknowledge pain.

"Men are taught to deny injury, as if they're wimps if they give in to it," says Stephen Pierrel, Ph.D., a clinical psychologist at Baylor College of Medicine in Houston. "So if we have an ache or some other symptom, most of us are ingrained to just tough it out."

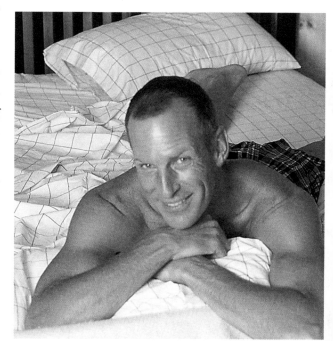

While that attitude makes for great sports headlines, it doesn't do much for your health. Aches, pain, and the like are warning signs that something's wrong, that you should stop what you're doing and get help. Now.

Unfortunately, men tend to miss or ignore pain and other signs of health trouble, and thus delay getting medical help. In a *Men's Health* magazine/CNN survey, 34 percent of men polled said that they wouldn't call a doctor even if they were having chest pain.

To keep you out of trouble, we've compiled a list of warning signs that many men either don't recognize or tend to ignore.

The Sign: Impotence

What It May Mean: Vascular Disease

Difficulty getting or maintaining an erection is often the result of reduced bloodflow to the penis, a consequence of blocked arteries. Because the arteries in the penis are so small and erectile dysfunction is an easily recognized problem, this sign of atherosclerosis may become noticeable earlier in the disease, says Marc R. Pritzker, M.D., an attending cardiologist at the Minneapolis Heart Institute Foundation. In other words, impotence can be an early warning sign that arteries in other parts of your anatomy, such as your heart and head, are also becoming blocked, raising your risk of heart attack and stroke.

What to Do

- See your doctor for a thorough evaluation, which may include an exercise stress test.

Men Who Won't Get Medical Help—And the Women Who Love Them

When the man in your life won't go to the doctor even though he clearly has a health problem, here's what you can do.

Make it about you. "Tell him, 'I love you, and I want you to go see the doctor for me. I want to be sure that you're around for as long as possible because I need you,'" suggests Stephen Pierrel, Ph.D., a clinical psychologist at Baylor College of Medicine in Houston. While men tend to ignore their symptoms, they're less likely to do so if they realize that their problem is your problem, too.

Remind him of his responsibilities. Men take pride in their roles as caretakers and providers. So remind your man that he won't be able to take care of or provide for you and the clan if he isn't healthy—or, worse, isn't around, Dr. Pierrel says.

Nix the nagging. "Nagging often pushes them even further away from what you want," Dr. Pierrel explains. Enough said.

Call anyway. If you think that he's in immediate danger, and he still refuses to get help, call 911. You'd rather have him alive and angry than the alternative.

- Follow your doctor's advice. If the test results confirm vascular disease, he may prescribe some changes in your lifestyle—a lower-fat diet or more exercise, for example—or drug or other types of therapy.

- Do not self-treat with prescription drugs such as sildenafil (Viagra) that may be available on the Internet. A thorough physical exam is in order.

The Sign: Unexplained, Profuse Sweating

What It May Mean: Heart Attack

Chest pain isn't the only symptom of a heart attack. Other common signals include unexplained and profuse sweating, pain or numbness in the arms, and shortness of breath. Some less-common ones are nausea and vomiting; dizziness, weakness, and fatigue; jaw, back, or neck pain; or palpitations.

Unfortunately, most men recognize just a few of these signs. In a Wake Forest University School of Medicine survey of 1,200 adults, respondents recognized just three on average. A common one—unexplained, profuse sweating—rang a bell with just one-quarter of those polled.

What to Do

- Call 911 immediately.
- While waiting for the ambulance to arrive, take an aspirin. Aspirin can prevent the formation of blood clots, which can further restrict bloodflow to your heart during a heart attack.

The Sign: Loss of Speech or Slurred Speech

What It May Mean: Stroke

Men are even less likely to recognize the warning signs of stroke—such as loss of or slurred speech—than the warning signs of heart attack, says Wayne Rosamond, Ph.D., associate professor of epidemiology at the University of North Carolina at Chapel Hill. "So they wait for the symptoms to get better," he says. In fact, stroke patients wait an average of 4 to 6 hours before going to the hospital.

Delay can be deadly. Potent drugs called thrombolytics, which can dissolve the blood clots that cause most strokes, thereby preventing brain damage, work only if given within the first 3 hours.

Keep a Ministroke from Causing Major Trouble

During a ministroke, blood clots form and obstruct bloodflow in the brain. Then they quickly dissolve, so there's no lasting damage. That's not the end of the story, however. A ministroke may be a warning sign of a major stroke to come.

If you've had a ministroke, your risk of a major stroke is 10 times higher than that of a person who's never had one.

I DID IT!

William Fair:
He's Beating the Odds
against Cancer

The hotshot head of urologic surgery at the famed Memorial Sloan-Kettering Cancer Center in New York City was feeling under the weather back in 1994. Way under. His wife noticed it. His colleagues noticed it. But William R. Fair, M.D., tried to ignore it.

Finally, his wife got him to a doctor. The diagnosis: colon cancer.

The cancer was surgically removed, but it had already spread. After a year of chemotherapy, another tumor was found. To fight back, Dr. Fair worked with a group of researchers attempting to develop a vaccine based on his specific cancer's cells. He also enrolled in the Cancer Help Program at Commonweal in Bolinas, California. The weeklong retreat taught him coping strategies, spiritual direction, yoga, and meditation. "I was changed by my experiences there," says Dr. Fair. "It was my first introduction to yoga and meditation."

Dr. Fair also contacted Sophie Chen, Ph.D., a research associate professor at the Brander Cancer Research Institute at New York Medical College in Valhalla. Dr. Chen had been working for years with a Chinese herbal combination called SPES (Latin for "hope") that was showing great promise against cancer.

"There are a lot of promising things such as SPES out there, and now that they're being studied, in 10 years or so we'll know for sure what they can do," he muses. "But I didn't have 10 years, so I just started taking it."

Dr. Fair may have that 10 years now. He says that CAT scans show progressive shrinkage of his cancer since he began taking the SPES. His personal experimental vaccine is still on the shelf, if he ever needs it.

"I definitely don't think it's the herbs alone," he says. "I personally feel that the dietary and lifestyle changes I've made are all equally important."

In addition to loss of or slurred speech, warning signs of stroke include paralysis on one side of the body, numbness, blurred or dimmed vision, or severe headache.

What to Do

- Call 911 immediately.

- Get in the ambulance and get checked at the hospital even if the symptoms subsided before help arrived. Stroke symptoms that come and go often signal a ministroke, which also warrants prompt medical attention.

The Sign: Frequent Urination

What It May Mean: Prostate Cancer

About three-quarters of older men complain of symptoms of prostate trouble, but only one-quarter ever get a simple blood test that can help determine whether the culprit is a benign enlargement of the prostate gland or prostate cancer.

Benign prostate enlargement, prostatitis (inflammation of the prostate), and prostate cancer can all cause the same symptoms: an annoying urge to urinate often, difficult or painful urination or ejaculation, blood in the urine or semen, or frequent pain or stiffness in the lower back, hips, or upper thighs.

A blood test called a prostate specific antigen (PSA) test can clarify, detecting prostate cancer early, when it's most successfully treated.

What to Do

- See your doctor.
- Get a PSA test to determine whether benign prostatic hyperplasia (medical lingo for benign enlargement of the prostate gland) or prostate cancer is the culprit. Both of these conditions are treatable.
- If your PSA test is negative, don't drop the ball. In its earliest stages, prostate cancer causes no symptoms. So make plans to get retested regularly.

The Sign: Unquenchable Thirst

What It May Mean: Diabetes

Roughly one-third of the estimated 7.5 million American men with diabetes don't realize that they have the disease. It's not that they don't have the symptoms of diabetes: an unquenchable thirst accompanied by the need to urinate frequently, unexplained weight loss, fatigue, blurred vision, slow-healing cuts or bruises, or recurring skin or gum infections.

Left untreated, diabetes can cause very serious complications, including blindness, impotence, nerve damage, even death.

What to Do

- See your doctor.
- Get a fasting blood sugar test, used to diagnose diabetes.
- If the diagnosis is diabetes, follow your doctor's advice. By making healthy lifestyle changes such as losing excess weight and taking your prescribed medications, you can keep diabetes under control and avoid complications.

CHAPTER 9

The Men's Health Companion

Solve six common men-only problems naturally.

Study after study shows that most men hate going to the doctor. The reasons why range from busy schedules to tough attitudes to fear.

If you're one of these men, you'll love the information we've compiled here. Granted, you still need to get checked out by a doctor to make sure your symptoms are not life-threatening. Once you know they're not, they may respond quite well to self-care.

This chapter will help you take care of six common health problems on your own. Use it well, and you'll gain personal control over your health and healing. Just remember, there are times when it is foolish and potentially deadly not to see a physician. Any time you have a symptom that persists, have a doctor check it out.

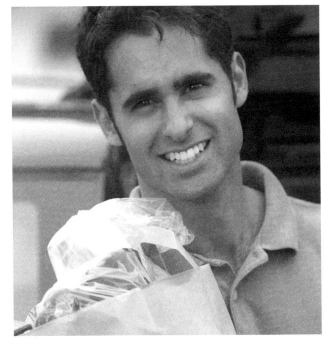

Baldness

Two of three American men develop some form of hair loss, and half are markedly bald by the time they're 50. The cause is androgenetic alopecia, the medical term for male pattern baldness. It accounts for 95 percent of hair loss in men. But it can be treated. Here's how.

Take some sage advice. In the old days, people often used sage extracts in hair rinses and shampoos. The herb allegedly had the ability to prevent hair loss and maintain color. Add a few teaspoons of sage tincture to your shampoo, suggests James A. Duke, Ph.D., author of *The Green Pharmacy Antiaging Prescriptions*.

Oil up. Using the Ayurvedic herbs amla and ashwaganda, you can make a preparation that stimulates hair growth, according to Partap Chauhan, an Ayurvedic physician in Haryana, India. Crush 1 ounce each amla and ashwaganda (available through mail order) into a rough powder. Combine the powder with 7 cups of water and soak overnight. The next day, boil the mixture until it's reduced by 75 percent. Strain it and add a small amount of sesame oil—approximately one-quarter the amount of the herb-water mixture. Boil again, until everything evaporates and only the oil remains. Cool, strain, and bottle. Some fragrance oils can be added at this time. Massage the oil into your hair and scalp twice a week.

Bladder Shyness

About 4 to 5 percent of men find that they just cannot urinate when they're near others doing the same thing in a public restroom, says Joseph Himle, Ph.D., assistant clinical professor of psychiatry at the

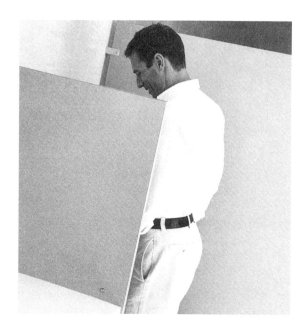

University of Michigan Medical School in Ann Arbor. Experts aren't certain why this happens, but Dr. Himle says that a combination of low self-esteem and general social anxiety—coupled, perhaps, with physical factors—may be the best explanation.

The good news is that bladder shyness can be overcome. These tips can help.

Practice. Using bathroom stalls and restricting your visits to the men's room to nonpeak hours only circumvent the problem, Dr. Himle says. He favors a strategy whereby a guy with a bashful bladder drinks lots of fluids, then visits public restrooms and repeatedly practices doing what should come naturally.

Start with an isolated bathroom, urinating 10 to 15 times for a few seconds each time during the course of an hour. Once you've mastered that, you graduate to a slightly more crowded restroom before eventually going on to conquer, say, a lavatory at halftime during the next Super Bowl.

Stay dry. If you're not trying Dr. Himle's tactic, then quaffing several brews or soft drinks at a ball game doesn't make much sense. It's your choice: Work on becoming comfortable enough to urinate in a public restroom, or learn to enjoy not drinking during events.

Delayed Ejaculation

In older men, delayed ejaculation may just be one of the consequences of aging, says Robert Birch, Ph.D., a sex therapist in Columbus, Ohio, and au-thor of *Male Sexual Endurance*. It can also be a side effect of certain medications, such as antidepres-sants, or the result of an injury to the nervous system. Some men find that they require a long time to ejaculate when wearing a condom be-cause of reduced sensitivity. Others are uncom-fortable with intimacy.

Whatever its cause, delayed ejaculation can be corrected. Here's how.

Drink in moderation. Alcohol is a depressant and can impede an ejaculation, says Dr. Birch. On a night that you're likely to have sex, try to keep your drinking to a min-imum.

Take This for Better Sex

If you've seen ads for a product called Venix and wondered whether it could do as it claims—boost your sex drive—the answer may be yes. Manufactured by Pharmanex, Venix is composed of several natural products, including ginkgo (*Ginkgo biloba*) leaf extract, cordyceps (*Paecilomyces hepiali mycelium*), and the amino acid L-arginine. Each of these ingredients has been shown to promote normal sexual function.

Ginkgo contains terpene derivatives that prevent blood platelets from clumping together, thereby improving bloodflow to the brain and other organs. Cordyceps has been shown in pharmacological studies to improve arterial blood supply, sug-gesting that it also promotes bloodflow to the sex organs. Other studies have shown that it has effects similar to those of the steroidal sex hormones, causing an increase in the weight of rabbit testes and also enhancing the sperm count. L-argi-nine, a naturally occurring amino acid, functions as a precursor to nitric oxide, a po-tent vasodilator. This dilation produces an increase in bloodflow that is necessary to the erectile function of the penis.

Venix is available in the United States by calling toll-free (888) PHARMANEX (742-7626) or by logging on to www.pharmanex.com. Venix is not available in Canada.

Junk the junk food. A diet heavy in saturated fats can, over time, harden your arteries, impeding bloodflow to the penis, perhaps making it more difficult to ejaculate, says Willard Dean, M.D., medical director of the Center for Self-Healing in Santa Fe, New Mexico. All men should try to get less than 30 percent of their calories from fat, and they should make more room in their everyday eating for foods like pasta and vegetables.

Look in the medicine cabinet. Some medications can make it more difficult for a man to ejaculate. These include some antihistamines, certain blood pressure medications (Diuril, Lozol, and Enduron), and some antidepressants (Prozac, Paxil, and Zoloft). If you're taking a medication and are having a noted difficulty in ejaculating, the two may be linked, says Neil Baum, M.D., associate clinical professor of urology at Tulane University School of Medicine in New Orleans. Ask your doctor about switching prescriptions, he says.

‖ Frequent Urination

Frequent urination is often caused by benign prostatic hyperplasia (BPH), or an enlarged prostate gland. As the prostate grows, it may compress the urethra, the tube through which urine passes. This makes urination more difficult. And when you do go, you don't completely empty your bladder, so it fills up more quickly and you need to relieve yourself more often. Another possible symptom: a lowered sex drive.

Half of all men over age 60 have BPH; by age 85, 9 out of 10 men are affected by the condition. Luckily, an enlarged prostate is not the same as prostate cancer, nor does it cause cancer.

If you're experiencing prostate symptoms, here's what to do for relief.

Supplement with vitamin E. This popular antioxidant may help protect against prostate disease, says Robert Cowles, M.D., a urologist in Atlanta. He recommends 1,000 IU a day. If you are considering taking large amounts of vitamin E such as this, discuss it with your doctor first.

Select selenium. Like vitamin E, the mineral selenium may help stave off prostate disease, says Dr. Cowles. He recommends 100 micrograms a day.

Try saw palmetto. Take 80 to 160 milligrams of saw palmetto standardized extract daily, recommends Thomas Kruzel, N.D., a naturopathic physician and professor of urology at the National College of Naturopathic Medicine in Portland, Oregon. Several studies show that the seeds from this palm tree are effective in treating BPH and its symptoms by blocking the conversion of testosterone into harmful dihydrotestosterone, Dr. Kruzel says. You should consult with your doctor regularly when using saw palmetto for treatment of enlarged prostate. In rare cases,

Examine Your Meds

If you have to urinate frequently because of prostate problems, try to limit the use of antihistamines and over-the-counter cold remedies, advises Robert Cowles, M.D., a urologist in Atlanta. They can cause a tightening of the bladder neck and the prostate and make it more difficult to urinate. This, in turn, makes you have to go more often.

people taking this herb have experienced stomach problems.

Opt for nettle. Taking 200 to 400 milligrams of dried root extract in capsule form three times a day continually works to shrink the prostate. Be sure to get dried root extract, and not dried leaves.

Cut back on fats and zinc. A study at the University of Athens Medical School in Greece found that men who ate a lot of butter, margarine, meat, and foods rich in zinc were more likely to develop BPH. Limit your fat intake, substitute olive oil for butter or margarine when possible, and avoid eating a lot of meat or taking supplements that contain zinc. Men who ate a lot of fruit ran a lower-than-average risk of BPH.

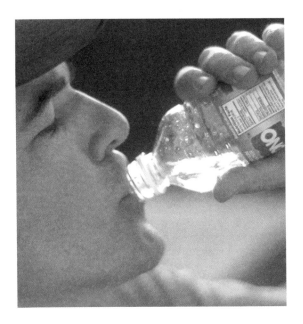

‖ Gout

In gout, uric acid—a by-product of the waste that your kidneys usually flush out of the body—builds up in your system and settles into the lining surrounding a joint, usually the big toe. This causes inflammation, swelling, and severe pain in the joint, possibly accompanied by chills, shivers, and a mild fever.

More than one million Americans have gout, and it's much more likely to affect men than women. In fact, three-quarters of those with gout are men, ages 45 to 50, says Doyt Conn, M.D., senior vice president of medical affairs for the Arthritis Foundation in Atlanta.

If you have gout, you'll no doubt want relief—fast. Any of these remedies may do the trick.

Drink water. Drink at least eight 8-ounce glasses of water a day to help flush the uric acid out of the kidneys, says Dr. Conn.

Double up. Bromelain, an enzyme found in pineapples, and quercetin, a bioflavonoid (a pigment in plants), are two natural remedies available in pill form at health food stores. "You should take 125 to 250 milligrams of each three times a day between meals when you experience a flare-up," says Devra Krassner, N.D., a naturopathic and homeopathic physician in Portland, Maine. "You can also add 1.8 grams of eicosapentaenoic acid (EPA) to this every day."

Flaxseed oil and fish oils are rich in EPA, which is an omega-3 fatty acid, a type of fat valued for its anti-inflammatory effects. Foods that are rich in EPA include green leafy vegetables, seeds (especially flaxseed), nuts, and grains. Some of the best seafood sources of EPA are anchovies, bluefin tuna, herring, mackerel, sardines, and all types of salmon except smoked. EPA is also available in capsule and liquid form at health food stores.

Call on Colchicum. "Colchicum is the homeopathic equivalent of colchicine, the prescription medicine that many Western doctors prescribe," Dr. Krassner says. "It may alleviate the acute pain of gout. Take two or three pellets of the 12C or 30X potency two times a day until the pain subsides." You can find this homeopathic remedy, which is specific to gout, in a well-stocked health food store.

Impotence

Almost every man fails to achieve an erection rigid enough for intercourse at some point during his adult life, says Drogo K. Montague, M.D., director of the Center for Sexual Function at the Cleveland Clinic Foundation. And for up to 30 million American men, getting and maintaining an erection is a persistent problem. Commonly known as impotence, doctors now call this condition erectile dysfunction. It can improve with some lifestyle changes—though you really should see a urologist to rule out a more serious underlying medical problem.

Lay off the beer or wine. Alcohol is a depressant that slows down your reflexes, including sexual ones. Limit yourself to one drink a day—which equals a 12-ounce beer, a 5-ounce glass of wine, or a 1½-ounce shot of

---

QUICK & HEALTHY

TOMATO-BASIL SAUCE

Eating more vegetables is one of the best ways to keep your blood vessels clear and supple, which will prevent problems such as impotence as well as heart disease. Yet few men eat as many as they should. This recipe gives you an easy and delicious way to sneak numerous veggies into your diet.

½	tablespoon extra-virgin olive oil
4	cloves garlic, minced, or 4 teaspoons prepared minced garlic
2	cups diced plum tomatoes or 1 can (14½ ounces) diced tomatoes
¼	cup tomato paste
¼	cup dry red wine or red grape juice
1	cup baby spinach leaves
½	cup sliced fresh basil

Warm the oil in a large saucepan over medium-high heat. Add the garlic and stir for 1 minute. Stir in the tomatoes, tomato paste, and wine or grape juice. Cook for 6 minutes.

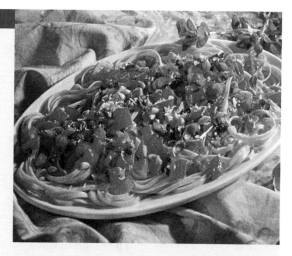

Add the spinach and cook for 1 minute. Stir in the basil. Serve over pasta and vegetables.

MAKES 6 SERVINGS (6 CUPS)

Per serving: 97 calories, 7.6 g protein, 12.4 g carbohydrates, 3.9 g fat, 0 mg cholesterol, 3.9 g dietary fiber, 118 mg sodium

Is Viagra for You?

As easy to take as an aspirin, sildenafil (Viagra) has quickly become known for its ability to restore a man's erections even after decades of impotence. In its first 3 months on the U.S. market in 1998, doctors wrote more than two million prescriptions for this "miracle drug," making it the most successful new pharmaceutical on record.

The drug works wonders for about 80 percent of men, stimulating bloodflow to the penis and jump-starting long-lost erections. But for nearly one in three men, particularly those with diabetes and other health conditions that damage nerves in the penis, Viagra may not help as much.

Viagra has other downsides as well. Doctors say that you should never use Viagra if you are taking nitroglycerin or related nitrate-containing drugs. When combined, Viagra and nitrates can cause a dangerous drop in blood pressure, and some men have died from this side effect, says Roger Crenshaw, M.D., a psychiatrist and sex therapist in La Jolla, California.

liquor—if you want to keep your erections as you get older.

Slice the fat. Dietary fat contributes to clogged arteries all over the body. So what's good for your heart is also good for your penis, Dr. Montague says. To stay potent, trim the fat in your diet to about 20 percent of total calories. If you eat 2,000 calories a day, that means you can eat up to 44 grams of fat, he explains. To get started in the right direction, read food labels, avoid fried foods, look for low-fat and fat-free products, and switch to fat-free milk.

Heart Disease Alert

Recent research has uncovered a completely different—and much more delicious—way to beat heart disease. Just add oil!

Heart disease, America's worst public-health enemy, is progressive, brought on in part by genetics and by years of unhealthy eating and too little exercise. Over time, poor eating habits can cause red blood cells to stick together, producing dangerous clots. They also cause cholesterol to line your arteries, narrowing the space that blood flows through and making blockages likely.

"Eating a heart-friendly diet is one of the most effective ways to prevent artery-clogging heart disease," says cardiac nutritionist Julie Avery, R.D., a registered dietitian in preventive cardiology at the Cleveland Clinic Foundation in Cleveland.

Exactly what to eat to beat heart disease has evolved. Experts once thought that a very low fat diet was all you needed. Now dramatic new evidence is showing quite the opposite. More fat, especially the right types of fat, is the way to go.

Here are the latest tips gleaned from current studies on how to eat to beat heart disease.

Take the Italian cure. Substitute olive oil for butter or margarine at the table, drizzle it on salads, and use it to replace vegetable oils in baking wherever possible. Buy only cold-pressed

extra-virgin oil; it retains more heart-healthy antioxidants than other forms.

Swap meat for fish. "I encourage everyone to trade some of their meat meals for at least one or two fish meals and one or two vegetarian meals each week," says Avery. Including fish is a great heart-protective strategy because fish

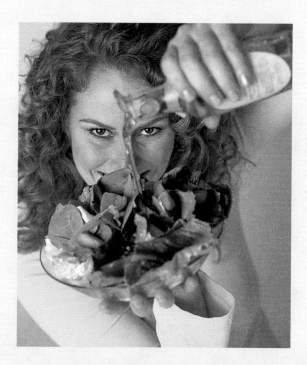

QUICK & HEALTHY
GRILLED RED SNAPPER WITH GAZPACHO SAUCE

If you've shied away from heart-healthy fish because you didn't know how to prepare it, now you have no excuse. Just use this delicious recipe.

4	teaspoons olive oil
1	slice French or Italian bread
3	small cloves garlic, unpeeled
½	cup coarsely chopped, peeled, and seeded tomatoes
½	cup coarsely chopped roasted red bell pepper, drained
2	teaspoons red wine vinegar or other vinegar
	Salt and pepper
4	red snapper fillets, ½" thick and 6 ounces each, with skin
2–3	teaspoons chopped fresh basil

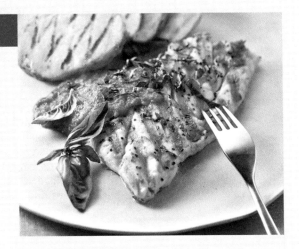

Preheat the grill to hot.

Heat 2 teaspoons of the oil in a small, heavy skillet over low heat. Add bread and garlic. Lightly brown the bread on both sides, then remove. Continue to cook garlic, turning occasionally, for 1 to 2 minutes, until tender.

Combine the tomatoes, roasted pepper, vinegar, toasted bread broken into pieces, and peeled garlic in a blender, and puree until smooth. Season with salt and pepper.

Moisten both sides of the fillets with the remaining 2 teaspoons of oil, and season with salt and pepper. Place skin side down on the grill and cook for 4 to 5 minutes. Turn and grill 4 to 5 minutes longer, until the fish flakes easily.

Place the fillets on plates, top with a dollop of sauce, and sprinkle with basil. Serve remaining sauce on the side.

MAKES 4 SERVINGS

Per serving: 248 calories, 36 g protein, 7 g carbohydrates, 7 g fat, 63 mg cholesterol, 0 g dietary fiber, 231 mg sodium

---

has much less total fat and saturated fat than most meat. Plus, cold-water fish such as salmon, tuna, and mackerel harbor another heart-disease fighting secret: omega-3 fatty acids. This special fat may lower blood pressure, keep blood from clotting, and buoy the "good" HDL cholesterol.

Dig into dark chocolate. An ounce of dark chocolate contains 10 times more antioxidants than a strawberry. Preliminary research shows that eating 1 ounce of chocolate each day increases "good" HDL cholesterol and prevents "bad" LDL cholesterol from oxidizing, which may lead to heart disease.

Linger in the produce aisle. Eat at least nine servings of fresh fruits and vegetables every day. Emphasize cruciferous vegetables such as kale, brussels sprouts, broccoli, and cabbage, which are a gold mine of antioxidants and other heart-saving phytochemicals.

Go nuts. Studies have found that those who eat more than 5 ounces of nuts a week are one-third less likely to have heart disease or a heart attack.

Drink more grape juice. The grape juice that helps prevent blood clots and oxidation of "bad" LDL cholesterol is made from 100 percent Concord grapes and is dark purple rather than red. To be sure that you're getting the good stuff, insist on seeing the words "100 percent Concord grape juice" on the label.

| natural
WONDER
TOMATO SEEDS
The yellow-jelly innards surrounding tomato seeds may contain a potent clot-fighting compound. This is important because clots can block blood vessels, leading to heart attack and stroke.

Grab garlic. Just one clove a day—or 300 milligrams three times daily—reduces the risk of a heart attack at least three ways: It discourages red blood cells from sticking together and blocking your arteries, reduces arterial damage, and discourages cholesterol from lining those arteries and causing blockages in them.

Reach for soy. Vegetable protein, especially soy protein, can help keep the pipelines in the heart open, says Mark Messina, Ph.D., a nutritionist, private consultant, and soybean expert in Port Townsend, Washington. Studies suggest that one of the

12 Foods That Stop a Stroke

Potassium-rich foods help stop strokes, which hit half a million Americans every year. This mineral also fights high blood pressure, something that 50 million of us have. Here are 12 super-rich potassium sources.

Source	Potassium (mg)	Calories
1 baked potato with skin	903	212
1 c prune juice	707	182
5 dried peach halves	648	156
1 baked potato without skin	641	156
1 c low-fat plain yogurt	520	130
½ c cooked Swiss chard	483	18
10 dried apricot halves	482	83
1 c orange juice from concentrate	473	112
1 banana	451	105
½ c cooked acorn squash, cubed	446	57
½ c cooked spinach	419	21
¾ c tomato juice	400	31

Tofu Made Easy

To easily prepare delicious and heart-healthy tofu dishes, use these tips from Reed Mangels, R.D., Ph.D., nutrition advisor for the Vegetarian Resource Group in Baltimore.

Keep tofu well-watered. Tofu is very perishable. Refrigerate fresh tofu for up to a week in a closed container of water and change the water every day. If you have kept tofu past its prime, it will smell slightly sour. Discard it.

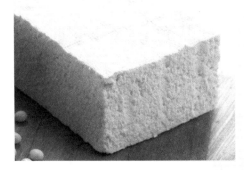

Marinate away. One of tofu's most characteristic traits is its plainness—that is, fresh tofu doesn't have a very strong flavor of its own. Take advantage of this blandness by marinating tofu in whatever flavor you savor. A soy sauce and ginger marinade is a natural, in keeping with tofu's Eastern origins. But think creatively. An olive oil–fresh basil marinade could be just perfect if you would like to stir those chunks of flavored tofu into spaghetti sauce.

Go eggless. A great way to disguise tofu is to make a mock egg salad. Use cubes of firm tofu instead of hard-cooked eggs. Mix with low-fat mayonnaise and a little mustard or add curry powder for color.

Try a change of texture. Freezing tofu gives it a chewier texture, closer to that of meat. Tightly wrap slices of tofu in plastic and freeze for up to 3 months. Defrost it at room temperature before you cook it.

ways it may do this is by helping lower cholesterol levels.

Get your minerals. Minerals such as calcium, potassium, and magnesium are crucial players in the heart-health scenario. In one of its lesser-known roles, calcium is part of a protein that helps regulate blood pressure. Potassium is believed to both prevent and help correct high blood pressure as well as keep your heartbeat steady. And, although there is less than an ounce of it in a 130-pound person, magnesium appears to be essential to healthy heart function, protecting that vital organ from heart disease as well as helping to control high blood pressure.

Stock up on Bs. Vitamins B_6 and B_{12} and folic acid keep a substance called homocysteine in check. Homocysteine is an amino acid that belongs in the bloodstream. But when the levels of homocysteine are too high, it contributes to blocking arteries. Some heart research has shown that if you don't get enough of certain B vitamins, homocysteine levels go up.

You can harvest plenty of folate (the natural form of the supplement folic acid) from dark green leafy vegetables and from legumes like peas and beans. For vitamin B_6, many unprocessed foods such as fish, whole grains, soybean products, fruits, and vegetables are bountiful sources. For vitamin B_{12}, your options are limited because it is found in red meat, and our hearts don't need the artery-clogging saturated fat that's part of that package. But fortunately, the nutrient is in milk, too. And if you drink the fat-free kind, you will get the benefits of B_{12} without the disadvantages of animal fat.

Eat more vitamin E-rich foods. Vitamin E acts as a scavenger, gobbling up oxygen-containing substances that make fats turn bad.

I DID IT!

Sarah Yerger: She Defied Her Family History

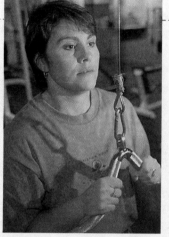

At just 26, Sarah Yerger knew she had inherited the traits that killed both her parents by age 50. A doctor's warning—and some good old-fashioned scorn—helped her save her life.

The cardiologist was blunt. After examining Yerger's mother one September day in 1995, he predicted that she would probably die of a heart attack within months.

"It wasn't the gravity of my mother's condition that scared me—she was an overweight, diabetic smoker who'd had heart problems for some time. Mom seemed destined for a heart attack like the one that killed my dad at age 49. What really frightened me? I was following in their footsteps. Though I didn't smoke, at 5 feet 4 inches, I weighed more than 200 pounds, ate all the wrong foods, and never exercised."

Within weeks Yerger joined a health club and began low-impact step aerobics three nights a week. That November, she joined Weight Watchers. She replaced her candy bars, fried-chicken-with-mayo sandwiches, cheese steaks, and beer-and-chicken-wing dinners with smaller, healthier meals. "Once I began measuring food, such as a cup of spaghetti and half a cup of sauce, I realized I'd been eating three times that, then loading it with cheese," she says.

By New Year's, she'd lost 2 percent of her body fat. She was down to 170 pounds.

In April 1996, just 7 months after the visit to the cardiologist, her mother died. "It was doubly painful knowing that if she had changed her habits, she'd have lived longer," she says.

Yerger stuck with her program and even began running. By Christmas 1996, she reached her goal of 135 pounds. "Every time I lace my running shoes or choose a celery stick over a candy bar, I prove that nothing is inevitable. Life is about choices, and I've chosen health."

Grapefruit Juice Warning

Don't take blood pressure pills with grapefruit juice. This combination can interfere with your body's absorption of calcium channel blockers (dihydropyridines).

While some people take supplements to get vitamin E, that might not be the best way. In one of the most convincing studies of vitamin E to date, researchers found compelling evidence that the amount reaped from a healthy, low-fat diet is enough to reduce heart disease risk in women. Post-menopausal women who ate the most vitamin E daily as real food—at least 10 IU—slashed their risk of heart disease by an astonishing two-thirds when compared to women who ate the least (less than 5 IU daily). Good vitamin E sources include wheat germ, mangoes, asparagus, and whole grain cereals.

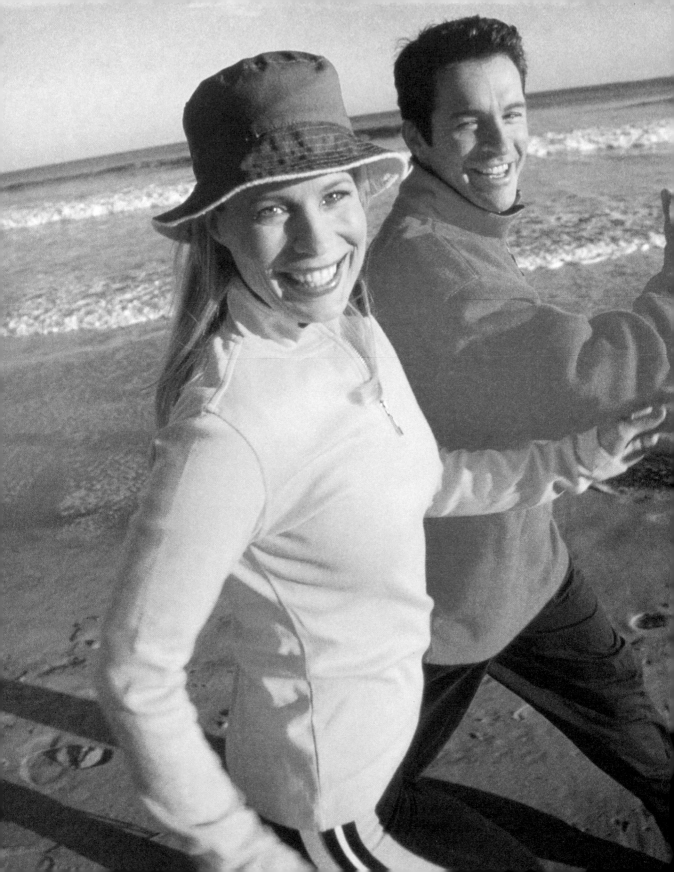

PART **FIVE**

Lose Weight, Love Life

Eat more, eat well—and still slim down with Prevention's *exclusive weight-loss plan.*

CHAPTER 10

The *Prevention* Diet

This 2-week program is so easy and satisfying, you'll want to stick with it.

You are about to embark on a 14-day adventure. By the end, you will be a new person in body, that's for sure. But you'll also be brimming with a new spirit—a spirit of accomplishment.

At the core of your 2-week program is the *Prevention* Diet, a mix-and-match eating plan that lets you choose your favorite foods from a list of delicious options.

For each of the next 14 days, pick a breakfast, lunch, and dinner from the following choices. Depending on your calorie goal, you can have up to three snacks a day. Each day you should be drinking two glasses of 1% or fat-free milk (100 calories each). And add a fruit or vegetable to any meal that doesn't already contain one. Also, eat at least one vegetable salad a day, made from your choice of lettuce, peppers, cucumbers, carrots, onions, broccoli, tomatoes, and 2 tablespoons of low-fat dressing. Men can have an additional two fruits and one milk daily.

Breakfast Choices
AVERAGE 300 CALORIES

- **Toast:** 2 slices whole grain toast with 2 tea-spoons peanut butter and 1 banana
- **Loaded Omelette:** 1 egg plus 2 egg whites, ½ cup chopped green bell pepper, and ½ cup chopped mushrooms; 2 slices whole grain toast with 1 teaspoon margarine
- **Egg-Cheese Muffin:** 1 poached egg and 1 slice reduced-fat American cheese on a whole wheat English muffin
- **Whole Wheat Breakfast Cereal:** Mix 1 cup cooked bulgur with 2 teaspoons brown sugar, 2 tablespoons chopped dried apricots, and 1 tablespoon chopped walnuts.
- **Cereal:** ½ cup high-fiber cereal with 1 cup fat-free milk and 1 cup fruit
- **Raspberry Smoothie:** Mix 1 cup low-fat for-tified soy milk, 1½ cups frozen raspberries or strawberries (no sugar added), ½ banana, ¼ cup light tofu, and 1 teaspoon sugar (or to taste) in a blender.

Lunch Choices
AVERAGE 375 CALORIES

- **Lentil-Broccoli Salad with Orange Dill Dressing:** To make the salad, toss 1 cup chopped romaine lettuce with 1 cup chopped broccoli, ¾ cup cooked lentils (canned are fine; just rinse and drain), and ½ tomato (chopped). To make the dressing, mix 1 tablespoon olive oil, 2 tablespoons orange juice, 1 tablespoon fresh chopped dill, ⅛ teaspoon salt, and freshly ground black pepper (to taste).
- **Fast Food:** Grilled chicken sandwich with extra tomato and extra lettuce, no mayo or

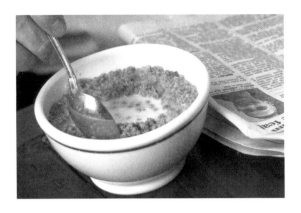

creamy sauces; garden salad with fat-free dressing
- **Sandwich:** Lean turkey breast, ham, or roast beef (3 ounces) on 2 slices whole grain bread with 1 ounce 50 percent reduced-fat Cheddar cheese, 1 cup arugula leaves, 2 slices tomato, and 1 tablespoon honey mustard
- **Easy Tuna Melt:** Mix ½ can tuna (packed in water) with 2 tablespoons light mayo, ¼ cup finely chopped celery, and ¼ cup grated carrot. Divide mixture between 2 whole wheat English muffin halves. Top each with ½ ounce low-fat Cheddar or low-fat Amer-ican cheese. Broil until the cheese bubbles.
- **Veggie Burger:** Serve on a whole grain ham-burger bun with 3 large romaine lettuce leaves, 2 thick tomato slices, and 2 tablespoons honey mustard; small bag of baby carrots
- **Pita Egg Salad:** Chop 2 cooked egg whites and 1 hard-cooked egg. Blend in ¼ cup chopped onion, 2 tablespoons light mayon-naise, 1 tablespoon mustard, and freshly ground black pepper (to taste). Cut the top off a 6½-inch whole wheat pita, then stuff with the egg mixture, romaine lettuce leaves, and tomato slices.

Dinner Choices
AVERAGE 475 CALORIES

- *Grilled Maple-Marinated Tuna:* Mix 1½ tablespoons maple syrup, 2 tablespoons orange juice, and freshly ground black pepper (to taste). Marinate a 5-ounce uncooked tuna steak in the mixture for 20 minutes. Remove from the marinade and grill or broil approximately 3 minutes on each side. Serve with 1 medium baked potato topped with 2 tablespoons low-fat sour cream and 8 large asparagus spears with 1 teaspoon margarine.

- *Trout Roll-Up:* Sprinkle 1 uncooked trout fillet (8 ounces, with skin) with ¼ teaspoon freshly ground black pepper and ¼ teaspoon salt. Top with ¼ cup chopped scallions. Roll from the small end, then wrap in foil. Bake at 350°F for 15 to 20 minutes. Remove the skin before eating. Serve with 1 cup cooked barley and 1 cup steamed green beans with 1 teaspoon margarine.

- *Mediterranean Pasta:* Heat 1 cup frozen broccoli spears, ½ cup white kidney beans, and ½ cup of your favorite pasta sauce in a microwaveable dish for about 3 minutes, or until heated through. Serve over 1 cup cooked linguine.

- *Grilled Chicken Breast (3 ounces):* Serve with 1 medium baked sweet potato topped with 2 teaspoons brown sugar and 1 teaspoon margarine, 1 cup cooked spinach with lemon juice, and 1 whole wheat roll with 1 teaspoon margarine.

- *Ginger-Cilantro Salmon Bake with Wild Rice–Broccoli Pilaf:* Coat a 9" × 9" baking dish with cooking spray. Place 3 cups chopped red Swiss chard in the bottom. Top with a 5-ounce uncooked salmon fillet. Sprinkle with (in this order) 2 tablespoons chopped fresh ginger, ½ cup chopped scallions, ¼ cup chopped fresh cilantro, and 2 teaspoons soy sauce. Cover tightly with foil, and bake at 350°F for 20 minutes.

- *Wild Rice–Broccoli Pilaf:* Sauté 1 cup chopped broccoli and ½ cup chopped scallions in 1 teaspoon dark sesame oil, 1 minced clove garlic, and dried oregano (to taste). When broccoli is still crisp-tender, blend in ½ cup cooked wild rice.

Snack Choices
AVERAGE 160 CALORIES

- *Trail Mix:* 2 teaspoons dried cranberries, 2 tablespoons raisins, and 2 tablespoons peanuts

- *Cookies:* 3 medium chocolate chip cookies

- *Veggies and Dip:* 10 baby carrots and 1 sliced cucumber with ¼ cup fat-free vegetable dip

- *Popcorn and Juice:* 3 cups low-fat microwave popcorn and 8 ounces calcium-fortified orange juice

- *Pretzels and Frozen Yogurt:* 1 ounce oat bran pretzels and ¼ cup frozen yogurt

- *Nuts:* ¼ cup dry-roasted peanuts

- *Yogurt:* 1 cup low-fat yogurt

- *Fruit Salad:* 1 sliced kiwifruit, 1 cup sliced strawberries, and ½ cup blueberries, topped with ¼ cup fat-free whipped topping

- *Brown Sugar Apple Bagel:* Mix chopped ½ apple with 1 tablespoon fat-free cream cheese, 1 teaspoon brown sugar, and ¼ teaspoon ground cinnamon. Spread on ½ whole wheat bagel.

Your 14-Day Program

Now that you have your eating plan in place, it's time to start your program. We've packed this 14-day planner with tips on working out, eating right, and staying motivated. This planner will serve not only as a daily reminder of your weight-loss goals but also as a record of your day-to-day triumphs and long-term progress.

Day 1

For Your Body

SET THE BAR LOW. What's the best way to stick with your commitment to exercise? Set the right goals. And in this case, think small. Wanting to run a marathon is great, but it may take months to achieve. That's too long before you feel successful. So think of lots of little goals, too, like "I want to do something physical every day."

For the Record

FOCUS ON FOOD. Since you're just starting out today, record everything that you eat. You can do it in the "What I Ate" section of the diary. Use the results to identify problem areas in your eating habits.

For Your Plate

PRIME THE PANTRY. Stock your kitchen with healthy foods—now! Your pantry should include such healthful staples as canned beans, whole wheat pasta and couscous, brown rice, white onions, canned tomatoes, low-sodium and low-fat broth, plenty of dry spices, balsamic vinegar, olive or canola oil, and fat-free cooking spray.

For Your Mind

MOTIVATE WITH MUSIC. Mood affects eating, and music affects mood. The upshot? If you're angry and heading for the cookie jar, stop at the stereo first. Try Pachelbel's Canon in D to soothe stress, anxiety, and a desire to eat.

Today's Diary

DATE:

What I Ate:

What I Did:

How I Felt (What Worked, What Didn't):

What I'm Proud Of:

‖ Day 2

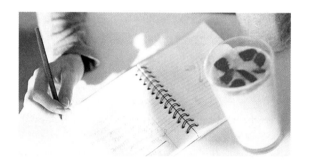

For Your Body

ALARM YOURSELF. If you're afraid you won't get out of bed to do your morning workout, here's a fail-safe plan: Set three alarm clocks—the kind that keeps beeping until you turn it off. Put one just outside the bedroom door so that you have to get out of bed to turn it off. Place another in the hallway and the third in the kitchen.

For the Record

COUNT 'EM UP. You may be shocked to find exactly how many calories and grams of fat you consume in a day—or you may be pleasantly surprised. Either way, use a nutrition guide to tally up your totals from yesterday's food list. Write them down in the "What I Ate" section of the diary each day to record your totals.

For Your Plate

MAKE PERFECT LOW-FAT PIZZA. Here's a trick to keep your low-fat cheese cheesy: Spritz it with a 3-second mist of cooking spray before heating it. This little bit of extra fat on the surface of low-fat or fat-free cheese makes the cheese creamy when it melts but without adding calories.

For Your Mind

ACCENTUATE THE POSITIVE. Don't beat yourself up, no matter how your diet and exercise plans go awry on any given day. If you did your whole workout yesterday but can manage only half of it today, you haven't failed. You've been active 2 days in a row, and that's great!

Today's Diary

DATE:

What I Ate:

_____
_____
_____
_____

What I Did:

_____
_____
_____

How I Felt (What Worked, What Didn't):

_____
_____
_____
_____

What I'm Proud Of:

_____
_____
_____
_____

‖ Day ❸

For Your Body

TAKE TEA WITH EXERCISE. Hydrating with green tea before you work out may actually boost your calorie-burn. The caffeine frees fatty acids so that fat melts away more easily. And the polyphenols (antioxidant compounds) in green tea appear to work with the caffeine to increase calorie-burn. (If you have high blood pressure, skip this tip.)

For the Record

HYDRATE WITH EIGHT. If you're like most Americans, you don't down the eight 8-ounce glasses of water that your body needs each day. Every cell of your body needs water to function, and a big glass can help keep hunger pangs at bay. Hydration is especially important when you're working out. Keep track of your fluid intake.

For Your Plate

OIL YOUR BREAD INSTEAD. You should already be eating whole wheat bread instead of white. The brown stuff has more fiber, which helps you feel full faster and therefore eat less. But what you put on that wheat bread is important, too. In a current study, folks who dipped their bread in olive oil ate an average of 52 fewer calories than those who used butter.

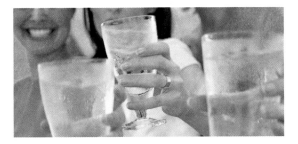

For Your Mind

LEARN TO LIKE YOUR LOOKS. Sure, you want to change your body, but you shouldn't hate it. Negative thinking can only sabotage your weight-loss plans. Stand in front of a mirror completely naked every couple of weeks. Find one body part that you like—even if it's your elbows! When you stop berating yourself, you'll shed pounds.

Today's Diary

DATE:

What I Ate:

_____

_____

_____

_____

What I Did:

_____

_____

_____

_____

How I Felt (What Worked, What Didn't):

_____

_____

_____

_____

_____

What I'm Proud Of:

_____

_____

_____

_____

‖ Day 4

For Your Body

SIT UP STRAIGHT. Hunching forward makes your belly look bigger. For a slimming effect that actually trains your stomach-supporting muscles to stay taut, sit with your shoulders back, chin up, and lower back supported against the chair.

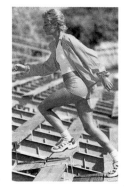

For the Record

TAKE A FEW FLIGHTS. Every little step helps burn calories and strengthen leg muscles. You burn 45 calories in 5 minutes of stairclimbing. Keep track of each flight you climb, and you may find yourself opting for the stairs instead of the elevator more often.

For Your Plate

SATISFY CRAVINGS WITH SMOOTHIES. To make a sweet shake that fills you up with healthful fruit, mix the following ingredients in a blender until smooth: 1 cup fat-free milk or soy milk, ½ frozen banana or ½ cup frozen mango slices, 1 teaspoon sugar, 1 cup frozen fruit (strawberries, pineapples chunks, or blueberries). Feel free to experiment by adding a touch of vanilla, cinnamon, or another flavoring to suit your tastebuds.

For Your Mind

SIDESTEP FOOD PUSHERS. When well-meaning friends or family members wave food under your nose and won't take no for an answer, try these replies:

- "Thanks, but I've already earned myself an extra hour on the stairclimber."
- "Could I take a little with me instead?" Once home, give it to someone else—or toss it.
- Distract them from the proffered dish by complimenting another: "I couldn't. I've already eaten too much of that wonderful shrimp salad. How do you make it?"

Today's Diary

DATE: _____

What I Ate:

_____
_____
_____
_____

What I Did:

_____
_____
_____
_____

How I Felt (What Worked, What Didn't):

_____
_____
_____
_____

What I'm Proud Of:

_____
_____
_____
_____

‖ Day ⑤

For Your Body

CREATE LEAN, STRONG LEGS. Try this easy do-it-anywhere move: Stand and lean back against a wall with your feet shoulder-width apart and about 18 inches away from the wall. Lower yourself in a slow controlled movement until your thighs are parallel to the floor, as if you were going to sit in a chair. Rest your hands on your thighs and hold for 15 seconds or as long as you can, then slowly slide back up the wall to the starting position. Repeat.

For the Record

STRIKE A POSE. We know you hate the thought of getting your picture taken right now, but posing for a "before" photo may help motivate you to trim down so you can take an "after" photo a few weeks or months down the road.

For Your Plate

GO SLOW. Mindful eating—concentrating on taste and sensation to make each mouthful an event—maximizes your food satisfaction and minimizes the chances of overeating.

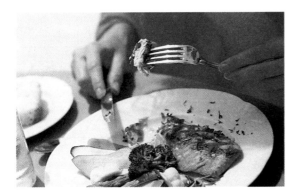

For Your Mind

BOUNCE BACK FROM SLIPUPS. Temptations and setbacks are a normal part of weight loss. It's what you do afterward that determines how quickly you get back on track. First, think back to what stimulated you to overeat or skip your workout. Then find a better way to deal with the emotions that drive you to eat.

Today's Diary

DATE:

What I Ate:

_____

_____

_____

_____

What I Did:

_____

_____

_____

_____

How I Felt (What Worked, What Didn't)**:**

_____

_____

_____

_____

What I'm Proud Of:

_____

_____

_____

_____

‖ Day 6

For Your Body

TO WALK FASTER, THINK POSITIVE. When a group of healthy people with an average age of 70 received about 30 minutes of positive subliminal messages, their walking speeds increased by 9 percent. To give yourself a similar boost when you work out, surround yourself with positive people and do things that make you feel good about yourself.

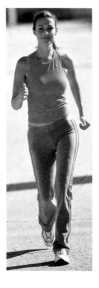

For the Record

UNCOVER EMOTION-DRIVEN EATING. Every time you eat today, write down what you're putting in your mouth and why. Are you hungry? Or are you mad? Or sad? Or bored? Charting your emotional eating will help you get a handle on just how much food you consume when you're not even hungry.

For Your Plate

CONTROL YOUR SPLURGES. Successful weight loss allows, even encourages, you to plan for an occasional indulgence in your favorite foods. In a current study of 24 obese women, those who learned how to deal with foods they considered a problem were able to lose weight steadily and keep it off. The women who just restricted their calorie intake lost weight initially but tended to regain it.

For Your Mind

DON'T FOOL YOURSELF. If you down a piece of birthday cake at the office, do you figure you'll eat less later? It's unlikely. When researchers fed 11 lean men a 250-calorie snack soon after lunch, they didn't feel more satisfied, delay dinner, or eat less later on. They simply tacked the extra calories onto their day's total.

Today's Diary

DATE:

What I Ate:

_____

_____

_____

_____

What I Did:

_____

_____

_____

_____

How I Felt (What Worked, What Didn't)**:**

_____

_____

_____

_____

_____

What I'm Proud Of:

_____

_____

_____

_____

‖ Day 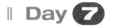 7

For Your Body

STOP SIDE STITCHES. That annoying pain in your side may be due to your preworkout drinking habits. One study showed that gulping down a quart of liquid immediately before exercising may make you more likely to get a side stitch than running on an empty stomach would. To prevent stitches while still staying hydrated, sip small amounts (4 to 8 ounces) of water more frequently over the course of ½ hour before you work out.

For the Record

GIVE YOURSELF A CHECKUP. Take a few minutes today to note how your body feels, from head to toe. Are your shoulders tense? Is your back sore? Do you feel as though your muscles are tight? How are your allergy symptoms? Do you get headaches often? As you continue with your workout program, you'll notice changes in your overall sense of well-being, and you can use today's notes as a baseline to see how far you progress.

For Your Plate

NIX NIGHTTIME SNACKING. People are particularly vulnerable to overeating in the evening. Experts believe that this may be because people don't get the same degree of satisfaction from food at night as they do earlier in the day. The solution? Go to bed earlier and get up earlier so you'll be eating at times when you get the most satisfaction from your food.

For Your Mind

TAKE THE ANXIETY OUT OF EXERCISING. If you're self-conscious about your body, exercise can be intimidating. To feel and look your best while working out, get some attractive fitness attire from your local sporting goods shop. If you're a woman who is a size 14 or larger, contact Junonia, a company that makes supportive, stylish activewear in these sizes for swimming, aerobics, and more. To request a catalog, write to 2950 Lexington Avenue, Eagan, MN 55121.

Today's Diary

DATE:

What I Ate:

_____

_____

_____

_____

What I Did:

_____

_____

_____

_____

How I Felt (What Worked, What Didn't):

_____

_____

_____

_____

What I'm Proud Of:

_____

_____

_____

_____

‖ Day **8**

For Your Body

HAMMER TIME. The hammer curl targets your biceps and the smaller muscles beneath them. The benefit? Quick results. Start by standing upright, feet shoulder-width apart, holding a dumbbell in each hand, with 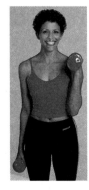 palms facing in. Bend your left elbow, slowly raising the dumbbell toward your left shoulder in a slow motion, as if you're hammering. Only your hand and forearm should move—don't twist your wrist. Lift until the dumbbell is nearly touching your shoulder. Pause, then slowly lower. Do 8 to 12 reps per arm for one to three sets.

For the Record

CHECK YOUR MEDS. Certain drugs, including antihistamines, diabetes medications, psychiatric medications, and steroid hormones, can lead to weight gain. Some stimulate appetite, while others cause you to retain nutrients, calories, or fluid. If you suspect that your medication may be causing you to gain weight, talk with your doctor about modifying your prescription.

For Your Plate

START THE DAY RIGHT. Contrary to what some folks believe, eating breakfast won't boost your metabolism. Skipping it, however, could lead to a 5 percent drop in your resting metabolic rate. Translation: You'll burn fewer calories at rest than someone who eats three or more meals a day. That small 5 percent can add up to a 10-pound weight difference in a year.

For Your Mind

MAKE LIFTING MORE UPLIFTING. Here are some tips to help you find the fun in lifting. If you like camaraderie, join a strength-training class at a local gym. If you prefer going solo, lift in front of a mirror and focus on your form. Still bored? Haul your weights to the living room and work out while you watch TV.

Today's Diary

DATE: _____

What I Ate:

_____

_____

_____

_____

What I Did:

_____

_____

_____

_____

How I Felt (What Worked, What Didn't):

_____

_____

_____

_____

What I'm Proud Of:

_____

_____

_____

_____

‖ Day ❾

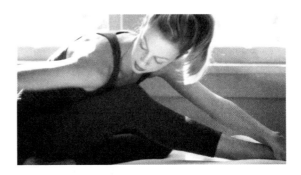

For Your Body

STRETCH IT OUT. To avoid pulling muscles or straining joints, make sure that you warm up and then stretch before you exercise. A brisk walk is a good warmup and cooldown for just about any type of workout.

For the Record

GO FOR WHOLE. Once you know what to look for on the label, track your intake of whole wheat bread, pasta, cereal, rice, and other whole grain products. (Your rice should be brown, Texmati, or wehani, not white.) Processed grains have less hunger-fighting fiber, and they turn to sugar practically before you swallow them.

For Your Plate

BECOME A BREAD DETECTIVE. Still trying to make the switch from white bread to wheat? It's not enough to choose a bread that's brown: The color may be due to dye, not fiber. Instead, make sure that the first ingredient listed on the package is whole wheat or whole grain flour. If it's not, it's mainly white flour. And don't be fooled by fancy names. Even if the first ingredient has a healthy-sounding name such as enriched flour or unbleached, unbromated wheat flour, it's still not whole wheat.

For Your Mind

QUIT COMPARING. If you have a buddy in the war on weight loss, don't get discouraged if he or she loses weight faster than you. Some people store calories more efficiently, and others burn them off faster. This doesn't mean that you won't reach your goal; it just may take you a little longer.

Today's Diary

DATE:

What I Ate:

_____
_____
_____
_____

What I Did:

_____
_____
_____
_____

How I Felt (What Worked, What Didn't):

_____
_____
_____
_____

What I'm Proud Of:

_____
_____
_____
_____

‖ Day ⑩

For Your Body

SOOTHE TIRED TOOT-SIES. A 10-minute foot massage can reduce fatigue and rejuvenate muscles. Wash your feet with warm water and towel them off. Next, move 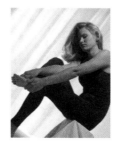 your thumb in long strokes from the heel to the base of the toes. Using firm pressure, make little circles all over the soles of the foot. For deeper relief, press your thumb directly into one point of the sole, and hold for a few seconds.

For the Record

FOR FEET'S SAKE, BUY NEW SHOES. If you're running or walking for your aerobic exercise, replace your shoes after every 500 miles. If you're not sure how many miles you're logging each week, take time today to measure your course by driving the route in your car and noting the mileage on the odometer.

For Your Plate

SAY YES TO CHOCOLATE—REALLY! Here's another way to avert a binge: Treat yourself (occasionally, of course) to a not-so-naughty treat. The following fudgy ones all have fewer than 100 calories apiece.
- Fat-free chocolate pudding (4 ounces)
- Two reduced-fat Chips Ahoy! cookies
- Fat-free hot cocoa (1 cup with 3 tablespoons whipped cream)
- Fudge pop
- Miniature low-fat ice cream sandwich

For Your Mind

TRADE FOOD FOR FUN. We all hit speed bumps that threaten to wreck our resolve. Before turning to food to relieve boredom, anger, or another negative emotion, do this: Make a list of fun things you like to do, such as call a friend, read a book, or take a walk. Then next time a bad mood strikes, try one of these activities instead of eating.

Today's Diary

DATE: _____

What I Ate:
_____
_____
_____
_____
_____

What I Did:
_____
_____
_____
_____

How I Felt (What Worked, What Didn't)**:**
_____
_____
_____
_____
_____

What I'm Proud Of:
_____
_____
_____
_____

‖ Day 11

For Your Body

EXERCISE WITH THE NIGHT OWLS. It wasn't long ago that experts advised against before-bed workouts, believing that they would prevent deep, restful sleep. Not so, say recent studies. In fact, for people who don't have sleep problems, nighttime exercise may help them nod off faster.

For the Record

PORTION YOUR PROTEIN. Do you eat enough protein? Too much? If you're choosing to have a little meat every day, make sure that the cut is about the size of the palm of your hand or a deck of playing cards—that's just 2 to 3 ounces. Even the smaller steaks at most restaurants are 8 ounces or more—that's three or four times as much as your body needs each day.

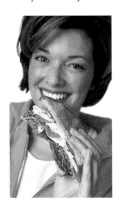

For Your Plate

SHUT OFF YOUR APPETITE. If you eat chicken, tuna, or some other high-protein food for lunch, you may eat less at the dinner table. In a Yale University study, women who ate a lunch of both carbohydrates and protein instead of carbs alone cut their dinner-time calorie intake by 20 percent. Experts believe that protein may trigger a greater secretion of cholecystokinin, a hormone that blunts appetite and makes you feel full.

For Your Mind

BOOST YOUR BRAINPOWER. Here's another reason to take a brisk walk today: Walking just 3 days a week translates into a 15 percent boost in mental functioning, which is substantial for such a small investment in time. Walking (and other forms of exercise) increases oxygen flow to the brain, which helps slow age-related declines in memory, the ability to manage multiple tasks, and the ability to shut out distractions.

Today's Diary

DATE:

What I Ate:

_____

_____

_____

_____

What I Did:

_____

_____

_____

_____

How I Felt (What Worked, What Didn't)**:**

_____

_____

_____

_____

What I'm Proud Of:

_____

_____

_____

_____

‖ Day 12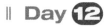

For Your Body

LOSE FAT, NOT BONE. In a University of Pittsburgh study, women who lost an average of 7 pounds also lost significant bone mineral density in the process. This isn't to say that you should stop dieting; extra pounds increase your risk of cardiovascular disease. Instead, you can protect your bones by doing regular weight-bearing aerobic activities (such as walking or running) and strength training.

For the Record

CALCULATE YOUR CAL-CIUM. You need at least 1,000 milligrams of calcium a day if you're a man or a premenopausal woman, and 1,500 milligrams if you're postmenopausal. Today, read the labels on your fat-free or low-fat milk, cheese, yogurt, calcium-fortified orange juice, and cereals and tally up your milligrams. Be sure to include the amount you get with your supplement.

For Your Plate

ORDER UP! Going out to eat doesn't have to be a diet disaster. In fact, you can order just about anything you want—as long as you don't eat all of it. Most restaurant portions are gigantic, and in one study, 26 percent of restaurant-goers admitted that they tend to clean their plates when they dine out. If you get a pasta dish, eat only 8 ounces (about the size of two tennis balls). A serving of meat should be no larger than a deck of playing cards. Have a serving of dessert the size of a yo-yo.

For Your Mind

TRY A FOOD-FREE MOOD BOOSTER. If you typically attack the snack cupboard when your mood turns foul, slip on your sneakers instead. Research has shown that exercise can improve your emotional state by triggering the release of endorphins, opiate-like brain chemicals that can make you feel good all over.

Today's Diary

DATE:

What I Ate:

_____

_____

_____

_____

What I Did:

_____

_____

_____

How I Felt (What Worked, What Didn't)**:**

_____

_____

_____

_____

What I'm Proud Of:

_____

_____

_____

_____

‖ Day ⓭

For Your Body

GET A LEG UP. Here's a good hamstring stretch: Lie flat on your back, legs straight out on the floor. Loop a towel or rope under the arch of your right foot. Pull your right leg off the floor—keeping your knee straight—until you feel a stretch. Hold the position 10 to 30 seconds, then release. Press your back to the floor throughout the stretch. Repeat three times per leg; do this five or six times a week.

For the Record

REVIEW YOUR WORKOUTS. Make sure that you're not lifting too much weight—or too little. If you can't do 8 repetitions at a time, your weight is too heavy. If you can do 12 easily, the weight is too light.

For Your Plate

SLURP SOME SOUP. Having a broth-based soup at the beginning of a meal can help you eat less. In one study, three groups of women ate a large bowl of chicken-rice soup, the same amount of chicken-rice casserole, or the casserole and a 10-ounce glass of water. In each case, the appetizer was made up of the same ingredients, but the women who ate the soup chose lunches that had about 100 calories fewer than the lunches the other women had.

For Your Mind

DON'T BE LISTLESS. If your resolve is already flagging, it's time to get out your pen and paper.

Close your eyes and take a few minutes to revisit what has brought you to this point in your life. Write down all of the reasons you want to slim down (not the reasons others think you should). Post your list on the fridge and keep a copy in your wallet. When your motivation wanes, give it a read and congratulate yourself for choosing a healthier life.

Today's Diary

DATE:

What I Ate:

_____

_____

_____

_____

What I Did:

_____

_____

_____

_____

How I Felt (What Worked, What Didn't):

_____

_____

_____

_____

_____

What I'm Proud Of:

_____

_____

_____

_____

‖ Day **14**

For Your Body

WALK THIS WAY. Want to kick up your walking workout a notch? Racewalking (basically, fast walking but with specific attention to form) tones your entire body as it revs up calorie-burn. To learn the technique, try Elaine Ward's video, *How to Walk Faster: Tips from the Pros.*

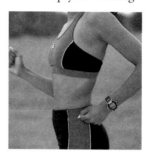

For the Record

GIVE YOURSELF A CHECKUP ... AGAIN. Remember those notes you made on Day 7 about how your body feels? It's time to reassess your physique. Is the tension in your shoulders subsiding? Are you getting more flexible? Do you have fewer headaches? Celebrate your better body with a massage or a long soak in a bubble bath.

For Your Plate

LOSE POUNDS, NOT BRAIN CELLS. Don't cut back too far on those calories, or you could wind up losing brainpower, too. In one study, some women who were on diets of 1,000 to 1,200 calories (half of their usual intake) for 15 weeks experienced a drop in iron levels and scored 50 percent lower on a concentration test than women with adequate iron levels.

For Your Mind

CAN THE COUNTING. If you simply hate to count calories and grams of fat, relax: You don't have to keep doing it unless you want to. By now, you should have a handle on what you're eating. Now, try to focus on moving more so you won't have to obsess about every bite you take. Instead of making dinner plans with friends, arrange "play dates" for tennis or swimming laps. And when your kids go out to play, join them!

Today's Diary

DATE:

What I Ate:

_____

_____

_____

_____

_____

What I Did:

_____

_____

_____

_____

_____

How I Felt (What Worked, What Didn't):

_____

_____

_____

_____

_____

What I'm Proud Of:

_____

_____

_____

_____

_____

CHAPTER 11

Outsmart Your Food Saboteurs

Survive any tempting situation—from huge restaurant portions to vacation splurges.

It's relatively easy to stick with a healthful diet if you never leave your house. If you feel a craving coming on, you head to the fridge only to be confronted by carrot sticks. Not much temptation there.

But go out to eat, and suddenly you're confronted with huge, fat-laden portions that fill you out more than they fill you up. And it seems there's a conspiracy to sneak calories into your food. Restaurant portions are humongous. Convenience-store fare is often anything but healthy. And the best foods served at a picnic are the ones swimming in mayo. Not to worry. Whether you're eating at a restaurant, fast-food joint, or amusement park, you can resist temptation—and even splurge a little—without gaining an ounce. Our tips will show you how.

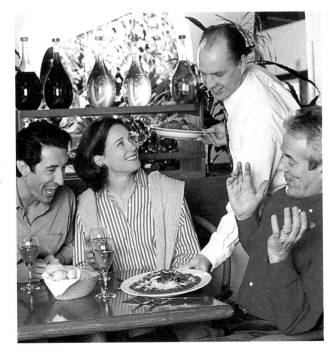

Dine Out without Filling Out

When it comes to dining out, there are plenty of ways to keep fun on the menu without padding your waistline. "If you put certain skills and strategies into action, it's possible to eat healthfully—and enjoyably—in 99 percent of restaurants," says Hope Warshaw, R.D., a nutrition consultant in Washington, D.C., and author of *The Restaurant Companion*.

Here's how.

Practice portion control. Use the three magic words: "Wrap it up." Ask if you can order half-, lunch-, or appetizer-size portions. Mix and match dinner salads, broth-based soups (like vegetable, beef vegetable, or chicken noodle), and appetizer portions of pasta, for instance.

Speak up—nicely. "Making special requests is essential to get foods as you want them," says Warshaw. And chefs are usually glad to oblige. A survey by the National Restaurant Association found that more than 9 out of 10 restaurants would, upon request, serve sauce or salad dressing on the side, prepare foods with vegetable oil instead of butter, and broil or bake an entrée rather than fry it.

Learn to say "fat" in five languages. French fries, Buffalo wings, and bacon

Restaurant Reality Check

How much is too much when you eat out? With our chart, which shows you common objects the size of sensible portions, you can easily eyeball the right amount to eat when you're served monster restaurant portions such as those below. Then watch those calories tumble! (*Note:* We calculated calories using sample portions in the USDA Nutrient Database.)

HOW MUCH YOU GET

Food	Restaurant	Calories
14-oz steak	Outback Steakhouse	1,213
25-oz pasta with meat sauce	Olive Garden	725
44-oz cola	McDonald's	555
2.3-oz chocolate chip cookie	Perkins Restaurant	318

HOW MUCH IS HEALTHY

Food	Serving Equivalent	Calories
3-oz steak	Deck of cards	260
8-oz pasta with meat sauce	Two tennis balls	232
8-oz cola	Yogurt container	101
Two 0.5-oz chocolate chip cookies	Yo-yo	138

cheeseburgers are fat bombs. But the word "fat" comes in other guises as well: "chimichanga" at Mexican restaurants, "carbonara" at Italian eateries, "crispy" at Chinese places, and "tempura" at Japanese restaurants. Wherever you dine, remember that items baked, broiled, grilled, poached, roasted, or steamed are typically lower in fat and calories.

Enjoy Your Vacation—And Don't Gain a Pound!

We know two women who are always on the road—for book tours, TV shows, and, sometimes, vacations. Yet they stay slim and eat healthy. One is Elizabeth Somer, R.D., author of *Food and Mood*. The other is Evelyn Tribole, R.D., author of *More Healthy Homestyle Cooking*. Both demand vacations with fabulous food. But they have some tricks to save calories—tips that you can use.

Refuel in 5. Don't go longer than 5 hours without eating, says Tribole, because then you're likely to overeat. "I become hostage to my stomach when I go too long, and then that extra cheesy sausage pizza looks totally enticing."

Drape your fridge. Drape a towel over the refrigerator in your hotel room so you can't see it, especially if it has a glass front. Your goal: to keep that fridge untouched. "Once I've broken the seal, I'm stuck, and I always eat something I don't even want," says Somer.

"Can" your food. Ask yourself, do I really want this? If the answer is yes, have it. "If the answer is 'No, I'm having it because my husband finished only half his ice cream cone and gave the rest to me'—you don't have to eat it. It's

I DID IT!

Penn Pollack: She Eats Out for a Living—And Still Stays Slim

Penn Pollack is a restaurant critic and must eat out five to six times a week. And we're talking full-course dinners. Yet, over the years, she's managed to stay slim, continuing to fit into her size 6 jeans. How does she do it?

Her first weight-control strategy is breakfast. She starts her day with cornflakes with 2% milk. Then she lunches at her desk on yogurt, crackers, and fruit.

On the nights when she eats out, Pollack takes along three or four friends to share the experiences—and the calories. "I only take three or four bites of each dish," she says. She also allows her companions to choose the higher-fat courses while she opts for the low-fat fish, chicken, or vegetarian. She often has fruit for dessert.

okay to throw food away," says Somer. "Better the trash can gets it than your hips!"

Describe and ask. At routine meals, keep the menu closed. Just tell the waiter what you want, then ask: "Can you get that for me?"

"At breakfast, I might say, 'I'd like two scrambled eggs, some sliced tomatoes, whole wheat toast, a glass of low-fat milk, and a big glass of orange juice. Can you get that for me?'" says Somer. "Be specific about what you don't want. Say, 'I don't want sausage; I don't want hash browns.' Otherwise, they bring it—and if it's there, you'll eat it!"

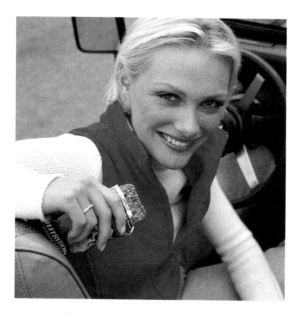

Expect the worst. If you're going to a zoo or amusement park, assume you won't find anything nutritious to eat, and take healthy snacks with you. Pick up some reduced-fat cheese, rye crisp bread, bottled water, and apples at a corner market. Instead of two waffle cones, Somer explains, you can have a waffle cone and an apple.

Complete a Road Trip without the Cupcakes

You've been stuck in the car for hours when you stop at a convenience store to fill up the gas tank and hit the restroom. Somehow you return with a bagful of chips, cheese puffs, and mini-doughnuts. Before you know it, you've added a few hundred empty calories to your hips.

During your next convenience-store run, keep these tips in mind.

Make it mini-meal size (250 calories) or less. To do that, always read the calorie count on the label. Many snacks are innocent-looking shockers, such as the Hostess Blueberry Hearty Muffin, with 590 calories—one-third of all the calories women need in a whole day.

Don't get snack amnesia. Compensate for your convenience-store snack by eating less later on. If you can't, try to avoid convenience stores by packing wholesome foods in a cooler before you leave on your trip.

Healthy Convenience-Store Picks

When you want a treat, these snacks have fewer than 250 calories and deliver nutrients that your body needs.

Snack	Serving Size	Calories
Crunchy Peanut Butter Clif Bar	1 bar	240
Planters Honey Roasted Cashews	1.5-oz bag	230
Kraft Handi-Snacks Mozzarella String Cheese	1 oz	80
Healthy Request V8 100% Vegetable Juice	10-oz bottle	70
Werther's Original candies	1 piece	20

Besides being low in calories, the best snacks have vitamins, minerals, and fiber—such as the treats listed in our "Healthy Convenience-Store Picks."

Indulge at a Picnic and Stay Just as Slim

Standard-issue, high-fat picnic fare usually consists of hamburgers, hot dogs, baked beans, potato salad, macaroni salad, pasta salad, deviled eggs, potato chips, brownies, blueberry pie, soda, and beer. Here's what to choose to keep calories under control without starving.

Entrée. Go for the burger, but hold the cheese and mayonnaise. A burger is higher in calories than a hot dog, but you'll be less likely to go back for seconds.

Sides. Scoop up ½ cup (approximately the size of a tennis ball) of baked beans for 160 calories and a whopping 7 grams of fiber, which will help curb your appetite. Depending on how they're made, the salads can have up to 240 calories per serving.

Snacks. Grab a deviled egg—just 90 calories each. A handful of potato chips has 60 more calories and offers little to fill you up.

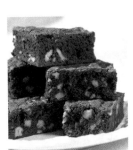

Dessert. Enjoy the brownie. A 2-inch square piece has about 115 calories. The pie: 360 calories.

Drinks. Diet soda has zero calories. Or how about a beer? Just make it a light—you'll save about 45 calories.

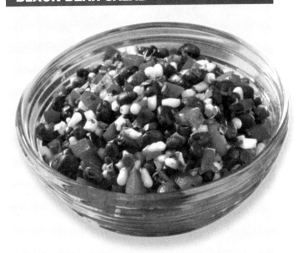

For a picnic dish that you know will be healthy, whip up a colorful black bean salad.

¼	cup red wine vinegar
2	tablespoons olive oil
1	teaspoon lemon juice
1	clove garlic, minced
2	teaspoons sugar
1	can (15 ounces) black beans, rinsed and drained
1	cup white niblet corn
1	cup chopped red bell pepper
¼	cup chopped fresh parsley

In a small bowl, whisk together the vinegar, oil, lemon juice, garlic, and sugar.

In a large bowl, combine the beans, corn, pepper, and parsley.

Toss the bean mixture with the dressing.

MAKES 9 SERVINGS

Per serving: 87 calories, 3.5 g fat, 3 g dietary fiber, 149 mg sodium

CHAPTER 12

Your Snacking Personality

Should you eat three or six meals a day? That depends on you.

For some people, snacking between meals curbs their appetite, so they eat fewer calories overall. But for others, snacking can substantially increase calorie intake and lead to weight gain. Which method works best for you largely depends on your snacking personality.

Snacking makes you fat when it begets snacking, says Stephen Gullo, Ph.D., author of *Thin Tastes Better*. Certain combinations of salt, sugar, and crunch can make it virtually impossible to stop at one or two bites.

And it's not just a taste thing. Snack foods can stimulate the appetite by their effects on our blood sugar, Dr. Gullo explains. Most snack foods are made with white flour, sugar, and very little fiber—even ones such as pretzels

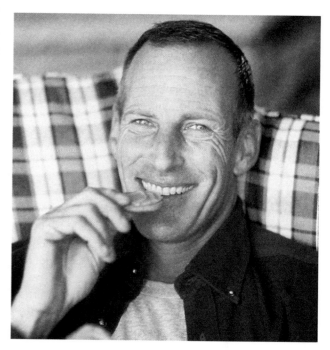

that we think of as healthy because they're low in fat. That combination of ingredients is just the thing to send blood sugar soaring and crashing, leaving hunger and the hunt for the next snack in its wake.

Get Your Appetite under Control

When you snack all day, you never let yourself get hungry. And eating out of hunger is critical to successful weight loss, says Marlene Lesson, R.D., nutrition director at Structure House, a residential treatment center for weight control in Durham, North Carolina.

Hunger usually means that your body actually needs the calories. But if you never feel

When Snacking Is Essential

Here are a few situations when a snack may be necessary.

- You're going to work out, and you haven't eaten in 3 or more hours.
- Your next meal is 5 to 6 hours away (unless that meal is breakfast).
- You didn't eat enough, and you're feeling real, physiological hunger between meals.

When you do snack, choose healthful and light foods, such as an egg white omelette, a cup of soup, yogurt, or a banana.

Who Should Try Three Meals a Day?

You may be an ideal candidate for the three-meals approach to weight loss if you:

- Skip one or more meals daily
- Snack all day
- Feel hungry all the time or have lost touch with your hunger signals
- Eat for emotional reasons
- Can't seem to slim down

hungry, you never learn to recognize your body's cues that it's really time to eat: You've burned off the calories from the previous meal, and it's time to stoke up your engine again. Eating three well-spaced-out meals a day will reconnect you to those all-important hunger signals.

Three Squares Can Keep You Satisfied

Here's how to go from the "nonstop buffet" to three meals a day without starving.

Plan ahead. Write down meals for the next few days or the upcoming week.

Eat till you're full. "My hardest job is getting clients to eat enough at a meal. When they don't, they're looking for a snack shortly afterward," says Lesson.

Don't skip meals. Cutting down to only two meals a day won't make you any slimmer. Your body knows how many calories it needs.

Meal Plan Comparison

Snacking Day

You may think you're eating healthfully by cutting out fat and sticking to mini-meals, but this may actually tally up to more calories. And the lack of fat and protein can leave you feeling hungry all day long, so you may be at greater risk of bingeing.

8:30 A.M. (breakfast) . . Coffee with fat-free milk and sugar
10:00 A.M. . . . . Fat-free muffin and coffee with fat-free milk and sugar
1:00 P.M. (lunch) . . . . . . Bagel with fat-free cream cheese and fruit salad
2:30 P.M. . . . . Bag of pretzels and bottle of sweetened iced tea
4:00 P.M. . . . . Fat-free fruit yogurt
7:00 P.M. (dinner) . . . . . Salad with fat-free Italian dressing
8:00 P.M. . . . . 1 pint fat-free frozen yogurt
10:30 P.M. . . . . 20 wheat crackers
1,926 calories, 21 g fat (10% of total calories), 15 g dietary fiber

Three Meals a Day

Here's how to enjoy heartier meals for fewer calories, so you'll lose weight without going hungry.

8:00 A.M. (breakfast) ½ cup high-fiber bran cereal with ½ cup blueberries and 1 cup fat-free milk
1 slice whole wheat toast with 2 teaspoons peanut butter
Coffee with fat-free milk and sugar

12:30 P.M. (lunch) 1 cup turkey-and-bean chili topped with 2 tablespoons low-fat grated Cheddar
¾ cup brown rice
1 cup steamed broccoli drizzled with ½ teaspoon olive oil and a spritz of lemon juice
Glass of fat-free milk
1⅓ cups fruit salad

5:30 P.M. (dinner) Spinach/feta cheese omelette (1 egg and 2 egg whites, ¾ cup steamed spinach, 3 tablespoons crumbled feta cheese cooked in 2 teaspoons margarine or oil)
1 slice whole wheat bread
½ cup low-fat frozen yogurt topped with 1/2 banana, sliced, and 1 teaspoon chocolate syrup
1,500 calories, 42 g fat (25% of total calories), 35 g dietary fiber

I DID IT!

Warren Prouty: He Changed His Snack Foods and Lost Weight

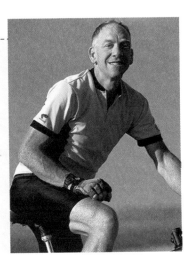

At 34, 305-pound Warren Prouty had three choices: die young, take blood pressure pills for the rest of his life, or lose weight. He chose the last option, in large part so he could see his two young daughters grow up.

In addition to exercising, Prouty learned to give up goodies by making healthy replacements. Instead of snacking on shortbread cookies or several pieces of coffee cake, he ate a pear, a peach, carrots, or fat-free yogurt. His healthy "trades" helped him lose 130 pounds . . . and get off his blood pressure medication for good.

When you skip a meal, your body demands those calories later, often when you're too tired to cook and junk food looks oh so appealing.

Go for balance. "Make sure your meals contain protein, carbohydrates, and a little fat," says Robin Kanarek, Ph.D., professor of nutrition at Tufts University in Boston. A tablespoon of peanut butter on your morning toast, tuna in your salad, or stir-fried vegetables instead of steamed helps you feel full longer.

Get some roughage. "Fiber is nature's appetite suppressant," says Dr. Gullo. Studies show that fiber keeps you feeling satisfied on fewer calories and helps keep blood sugar on an even keel, which staves off hunger. For breakfast, that means 100 percent whole grain breads and waffles and bran cereals. The rest of the day, make it a point to eat more 100 percent whole grain breads, whole wheat pasta, barley, beans, fruits, and vegetables.

Make it easy. Preparing dinner may seem overwhelming if you haven't done it in a while or need to whip something together after work. Use prewashed greens and prewashed, cut vegetables and fruit; prepared chicken; canned beans; scrambled eggs; and other easy foods.

Clean out your cupboards. "Get the right foods in the house and the wrong ones out," says Dr. Gullo. This includes tossing out low-fat cookies and crackers, even health-food-store versions, which are still loaded with calories. Worried about your kid's snack attacks? Hey, what's sweeter than a banana or a plum? You're not depriving your kids; in fact, you're helping them grow up with healthy eating habits.

Think pleasure, not deprivation. When you sit down to breakfast, lunch, or dinner, choose foods you really love.

CHAPTER 13

Burn Calories in Your Sleep

Learn the secrets of boosting a sluggish metabolism naturally.

Sometimes it seems as if you're doing everything right. You're eating 1,500 or fewer calories a day. You're walking every morning and every night. Yet you're hungry 24-7. And every time you get on the scale, you haven't lost an ounce.

The culprit: a sluggish metabolism. The good news is that you can kick-start your metabolism into high gear with the right combination of diet and exercise. In many cases, eating a little *more* of the right foods and doing a little *less* of the wrong types of exercise is all you need. You see, many people starve themselves, which slows the metabolism and sets them up for bingeing. They also overdo aerobic exercise, which only burns calories while they're actually in motion.

Yet by filling up with metabolism-boosting foods and building muscle

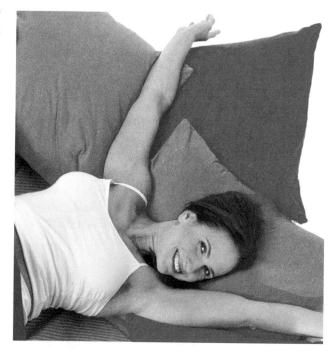

SALSA BEEF PATTIES

This naturally spicy dish is just what you need to rev up your sluggish metabolism.

1	**pound ground eye round**
¼	**teaspoon ground black pepper**
3	**plum tomatoes, finely chopped**
1	**jarred or freshly roasted red bell pepper, finely chopped (see note)**
2	**tablespoons finely chopped red onion**
1	**tablespoon finely chopped fresh cilantro**
1–2	**teaspoons finely chopped jalapeño chile pepper (wear plastic gloves when handling)**
4	**whole wheat buns, split**
	Romaine lettuce leaves

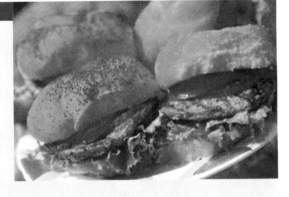

Preheat the oven to 450°F.

Form the eye round into 4 patties ½" thick. Season with the black pepper. Place on a broiler pan. Bake for 8 minutes. Turn and bake for 8 to 10 minutes longer, or until no longer pink in the center.

To make the salsa, mix the tomatoes, bell pepper, onion, and cilantro in a small bowl. Stir in the jalapeño pepper to taste.

Line the bun bottoms with the lettuce leaves and spoon on half of the salsa. Place the burgers on the salsa. Add the remaining salsa and the bun tops.

MAKES 4

Per serving: 356 calories, 26 g protein, 22 g carbohydrates, 18 g fat, 68 mg cholesterol, 3 g dietary fiber, 323 mg sodium

Note: Blacken a red pepper on all sides under the broiler. Wrap it in foil and set aside until cool enough to handle. Remove and discard the charred skin, seeds, and inner membranes. Chop the flesh.

with weight training, you'll create a calorie incinerator that gobbles up fat cells even while you sleep.

Metabolism-Boosting Foods

Research shows that the following foods can fire up your metabolism as well as slash hunger pangs, helping you to lose the weight you want.

Spicy food. A few small studies from Japan have shown that eating a fiery red-pepper-spiced meal may boost metabolism up to 30 percent. One downside: The studies used a lot of red pepper—between 5 and 6 teaspoons per meal.

Green tea. In a study from Switzerland, 6 out of 10 men who took a green tea supplement (the equivalent of 1 cup of green tea) three times a day with their meals burned about 80 more calories during the following 24 hours

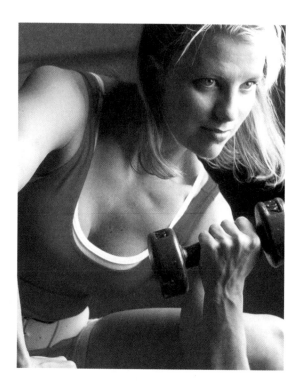

than those who took a caffeine pill or a placebo. The researchers believe that flavonoids in the green tea were responsible for the metabolism boost.

Coffee. The amount of caffeine (about 135 milligrams) in an 8-ounce cup of brewed coffee is enough to raise your metabolism for more than 2 hours. Drinking it before a workout may give you an extra kick. Caffeine may help free stored fat, so your body can burn it for energy as you exercise. (If you have high blood pressure, avoid caffeine before exercising.)

Metabolism-Boosting Exercise

Aerobic exercise can burn calories while you're in motion, but it won't help you burn calories in your sleep. For that, you need strength training, and that's why dumbbells and muscles are your metabolism's best friends. Weight lifting builds muscles, which then rev up your metabolism. Each pound of muscle burns up to 20 times more calories than each pound of fat, even when you're curled up with a book.

"After age 40, women start losing half a pound of muscle a year," says Wayne L. Westcott, Ph.D., fitness research director for the South Shore YMCA in Quincy, Massachusetts. "During menopause, that loss may jump to a pound a year. If you don't do something to put that calorie-burning muscle back on, it's very difficult to lose and maintain weight."

To get started, try the following circuit workout, which combines heart-thumping aerobic exercises with muscle-building strength training. Two days a week, do two sets of exercises for your upper body (see "Upper Body

Step It Up

No time to exercise today? Take the stairs instead of the elevator or escalator wherever you go. It's usually just as fast, you don't have to stand around waiting, and it burns 45 calories in just 5 minutes.

I DID IT!

Dinah Burnette: She Lost 100 Pounds— And Got into Her Little Black Dress

For many years, Dinah Burnette blamed her panic attack medication as she grew to a size 24. It wasn't until 1996—when she saw her graduation snapshots—that she realized how serious her problem had become. "I was beaming at the camera, but all I saw when I looked at the photos was 245 pounds stuffed into a size 24 dress. That's when I realized my medicine wasn't making me fat. I was."

To turn things around, she began drinking a daily gallon of water, eating a Lean Cuisine for lunch, and ending the day with a salad and fruit. She also began walking. At the end of each walk, her legs, feet, and back ached.

"To get through the hard times, I turned to my closet. There, my favorite black dress hung, waiting for me. Although that size 10 wouldn't begin to fit over my hips then, I knew that someday I'd wear it again," says Burnette.

To kick-start her metabolism, she started eating more, too. "I began each day with a slice of whole grain bread, a box of raisins, and a glass of fat-free milk flavored with a little instant breakfast mix.

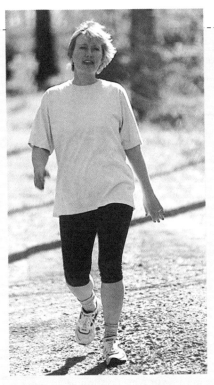

Throughout the day, I'd snack on fruit, low-fat yogurt, cereal, or raw veggies," she says.

Within 6 months, she'd lost 50 pounds and was down to a size 16. Exactly 1 year later, Burnette hit her goal: 144 pounds. "I'm still on the medicine, but at just half the dose. And the black dress? It's just a smidgen too big," she says.

Circuit" on page 138). Another 2 days, do the same for your lower body (see "Lower Body Circuit" on page 139). Use a weight heavy enough that you can lift it only 10 to 15 times before fatigue sets in. Then do 10 to 15 repetitions of each exercise. Between sets, do 2½ minutes of aerobic activity (stationary bicycling, treadmill walking, jumping rope, doing a snippet from an exercise video, marching in place, climbing stairs—anything you like).

‖ Upper Body Circuit

1. Chest press. Lying on a bench, hold the dumbbells end to end just above chest height, with your elbows pointing out and toward the floor. Press the dumbbells up, extending your arms. Hold, then lower.

2. Biceps curl. Hold the dumbbells at your sides, palms facing forward. Keeping your elbows at your sides, lift the dumbbells toward your chest. Hold, then lower.

3. Shoulder press. Start with the dumbbells at shoulder height, palms facing in. Press the dumbbells straight up overhead, then lower.

4. Bent-over row. Place your left knee and hand on a bench, keeping your back flat. Holding a dumbbell in your right hand, let your arm hang straight down with the palm facing the bench. Pull the dumbbell up toward your chest. Hold, then lower. Complete one set, then repeat with your left side.

5. Lying triceps extension. Lying on a mat, hold the dumbbells with your palms facing each other. Start with your arms extended upward and angled back about 30 degrees toward your head. Bending at the elbows, slowly lower the weights to either side of your head. Don't move your upper arms. Hold, then slowly raise.

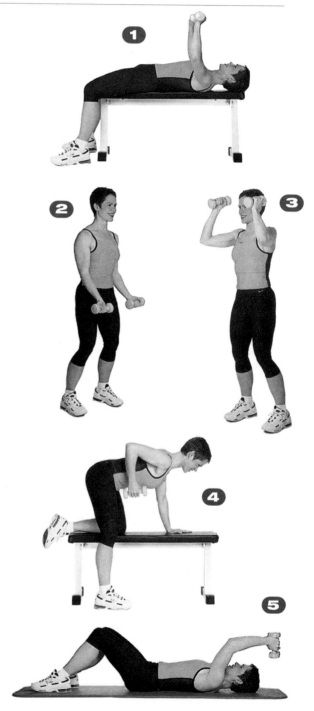

‖ Lower Body Circuit

1. Opposite arm and leg raise.
Get down on your hands and knees. Slowly raise and straighten your left arm and right leg off the floor as high as is comfortable, but don't arch your back. Hold, then lower. Repeat with your right arm and left leg.

2. Lunge. Standing with your feet together, take one big step back with your left leg. Plant your left foot, then slowly lower your left knee toward the floor. Your right knee should be at a 90-degree angle. Push off with your left foot, then return to the starting position. Repeat with your right leg. (To get more out of this exercise, hold dumbbells.)

3. Stepup. Using an aerobic step or regular step and holding dumbbells, step up with your left foot, followed by your right, so that both feet are on the step. Then step down with the right foot, followed by the left. Repeat, starting with the right foot.

4. Half squat. Stand in front of a chair with no armrests. Hold the dumbbells down by your sides, with your palms facing in. Keeping your back straight, bend at the knees and hips as though you were sitting down. (Don't let your knees move forward over your toes.) Stop just shy of sitting, then stand back up.

5. Abdominal crunch. Lie on your back with your knees bent and your feet flat on the floor. Place your hands loosely behind your head. Slowly curl your shoulders about 30 degrees off the floor. Hold, then lower.

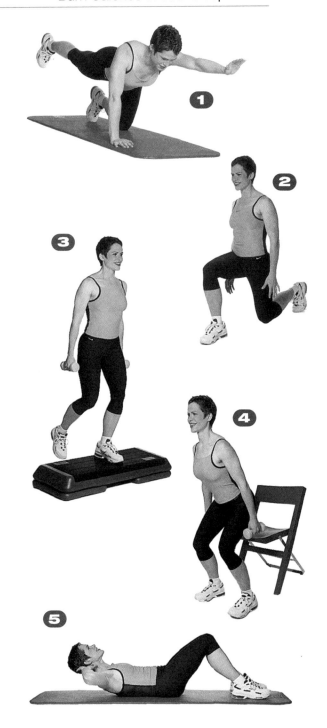

CHAPTER **14**

Guarantee
Your Success

Battling against dietary downfalls? Use them to
your advantage and lose the weight you want.

Most people have a food that—no matter what—they simply will not
give up. Here's the good news: you don't have to give up your favorite foods to lose
weight. Indeed, for many people, abolishing most-loved foods is the fastest route to
weight-loss failure.

That's why we're going to show you exactly how to incorporate the four most highly
craved foods into your everyday
meals—and still shed pounds. Whether
you love meat and potatoes, fast-food
hamburgers with fries, chips and dip,
or Death By Chocolate, we have an
eating plan for you. You don't have to
give up your favorite foods. These
eating plans will show you how to cut
calories elsewhere in your diet to save
room for the foods you love.

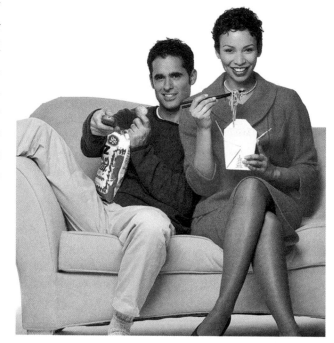

140

QUICK & HEALTHY
GUILT-FREE SCALLOPED POTATOES

Heavy cream is what makes this dish decadent. But who needs it, when you can get the same rich flavor—without all the fat—by combining fat-free half-and-half and 1% milk?

1	**tablespoon olive oil**
2	**tablespoons all-purpose flour**
1	**cup fat-free half-and-half**
¾	**cup 1% milk**
2	**cloves garlic, thinly sliced**
1	**teaspoon salt**
1½	**pounds baking potatoes, thinly sliced**

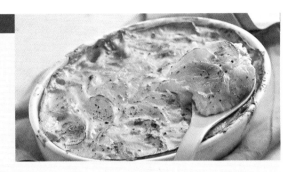

Preheat the oven to 375°F. Lightly coat an 8" × 8" baking dish with cooking spray.

Heat the oil in a medium saucepan over medium heat. Whisk in the flour and cook for 1 minute. Whisk in the half-and-half, milk, garlic, and salt.

Add the potatoes and cook until boiling, about 10 minutes. Pour the mixture into the prepared baking dish and cover it with foil.

Bake for 40 minutes. Uncover and bake for 7 to 10 minutes longer, until bubbly.

MAKES 6 SERVINGS

Per serving: 153 calories, 5 g protein, 26 g carbohydrates, 3 g fat, 1 mg cholesterol, 0 g dietary fiber, 419 mg sodium

‖ Meat and Potatoes

To continue to eat the comfort foods you grew up with, you must prepare them with fewer calories. Start with smart choices. Fatty cuts of red meat such as prime rib, T-bone, and filet mignon average 340 calories per 3-ounce serving. By comparison, their leaner cousins—top round, sirloin, and London broil—weigh in at 240 calories for the same-size portion. Grill or sauté them in olive oil spray instead of butter to cut calories even further.

For variety, try pork tenderloin or tuna steak as hearty red-meat substitutes. And explore other side dishes such as sweet potatoes and whole grain rice or pasta. They have the same starchy feel as potatoes, but they boost your fiber intake to fill you up faster.

Here's a sample 1-day comfort foods menu that supplies 1,530 calories and 51 grams of fat.

BREAKFAST
1 cup bran flakes
½ cup 1% milk
½ cup blueberries

LUNCH
Ham sandwich made with 1 ounce reduced-fat Swiss cheese, 2 ounces turkey ham, 1 roasted red bell pepper, romaine lettuce, and 2 slices whole wheat bread
½ cup macaroni salad (For fewer calories, ask if your deli prepares low-fat or fat-free side dishes.)
1 medium banana

DINNER

1 cup tomato soup made with 1% milk

3 ounces sautéed steak with garlic and cremini mushrooms (If you stick to the 3-ounce serving size, you can eat meat most days of the week.)

1 serving Guilt-Free Scalloped Potatoes (see page 141)

1 cup steamed broccoli

SNACK

1 apple

12 potato chips (Having a piece of fruit along with the chips can stop you from eating the whole bag.)

‖ Fast Food

Drive-thru food is great because it's quick and it tastes good. But there are ways to get the "fast" without the fat. Many burger places offer grilled chicken sandwiches and salad bars. If fried chicken is your weakness, picking off the breading strips the calories while retaining the flavor, says Susan

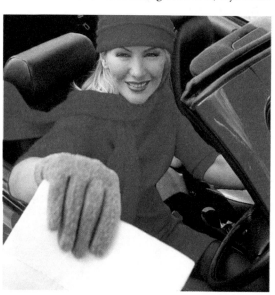

McQuillan, R.D., a registered dietitian in New York City. Overall, sub shops are a pretty safe bet—if you go easy on the mayo.

But when you just can't shake the craving, it's perfectly fine to hit your local hot dog stand or burger joint—just mini-size your meal.

Here's a sample 1-day grab-on-the-go menu that supplies 1,739 calories and 56 grams of fat.

BREAKFAST

8 ounces fat-free plain yogurt

⅓ cup strawberries

1 slice whole wheat toast with 1 tablespoon fruit spread

LUNCH

1 fast-food hamburger

1 small order fast-food french fries

12 ounces cola

DINNER

3 fish sticks, frozen

½ cup spaghetti with marinara sauce tossed with ½ cup cooked spinach and 2 tablespoons grated Parmesan cheese

1 whole wheat roll

SNACK

1 banana

4 ounces orange juice

‖ Junk Food

The trick to slimming down with junk food is to avoid eating the whole bag. You can get instant portion control by buying single-serving sizes of chips, sugary cereals, or candy bars.

Also choose "healthier" junk foods: flavored oatmeal instead of sugary cereals, a burrito instead of a hot dog, or toasted pita crisps and hummus instead of chips and dip.

Use this sample 1-day menu (1,560 calories, 52 grams of fat) to enjoy both sweet- and salty-tasting junk foods throughout the day.

BREAKFAST

½ grapefruit
1 cup oatmeal
½ cup 1% milk

LUNCH

Turkey sandwich made with 2 ounces turkey breast; 1 tablespoon light mayonnaise; ½ tomato, sliced; romaine lettuce; and 2 slices whole grain bread
½ cup corn chips

DINNER

2 beef burritos, frozen (Microwave and eat one burrito at a time. After the first, you may decide not to go back for seconds.)
½ cup corn kernels mixed with ½ cup sliced red bell pepper

QUICK & HEALTHY
CHOCOLATE INDULGENCE

This moist cake gives you a powerful chocolate taste with very little fat.

4	squares (4 ounces) semisweet chocolate
⅓	cup unsweetened cocoa powder
¾	cup sugar
½	cup evaporated fat-free milk
2	large egg yolks
½	teaspoon vanilla extract (optional)
3	large egg whites (room temperature)
¼	cup all-purpose flour
½	teaspoon baking powder
12	strawberries

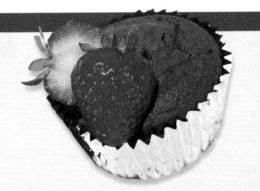

Preheat the oven to 350°F. Line a 12-cup muffin pan with foil. Place the chocolate in a large microwaveable bowl. Microwave on high for 2 minutes to melt. Stir until smooth. Set aside.

In a small saucepan, whisk together the cocoa and ½ cup of the sugar. Whisk in the milk. Cook for 2 minutes over medium heat, whisking constantly, until smooth. Stir the cocoa mixture into the melted chocolate. Stir in the yolks and vanilla extract (if using).

In a large bowl, beat the egg whites at medium speed until foamy. Gradually beat in the remaining ¼ cup sugar. Increase the speed to high and beat just until stiff. Use a rubber spatula to fold the egg whites into the chocolate mixture one-third at a time. Fold in the flour and baking powder.

Divide the batter evenly among the muffin cups. Bake for 20 to 22 minutes, or until a toothpick inserted into the center comes out clean. Cool.

Top each cake with a strawberry.

MAKES 12

Per serving: 133 calories, 4 g protein, 24 g carbohydrates, 4 g fat, 36 mg cholesterol, 1 g dietary fiber, 43 mg sodium

SNACK

1 jelly doughnut (Smaller doesn't always mean better. One cream-filled doughnut has fewer calories than 4 doughnut holes.)

1 cup 1% milk

‖ Dessert

You can indulge your sweet tooth at every meal. Since most of these foods are naturally sweet, you won't be going overboard on sugar. Try this sample menu (1,644 calories, 45 grams of fat).

⌐ I DID IT!

Matt Salmon:
From Marathon Eater
to Marathon Runner

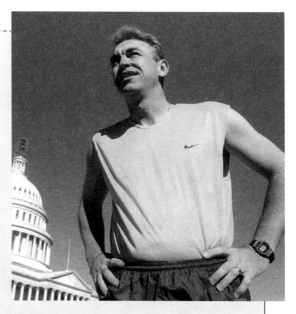

When Congressman Matt Salmon's political career skyrocketed, so did his waistline—until he decided to run for something other than election.

Each political dinner, fund-raiser, and charity event added another notch to Congressman Salmon's belt. Things got really bad in 1994 when he won a seat in the U.S. House of Representatives. Every week he traveled to Washington, which meant that family meals were out and Big Macs were in. And when he got famished between legislative hearings, he'd wolf down anything in sight—usually cookies or a piece of cake.

After coming across old photographs of his younger, fitter self, Salmon decided to take action. "First, I dealt with the constant political dinners and airplane meals by requesting low-fat or vegetarian meals. Next, I cut out high-fat desserts. That was hard, but I was no longer willing to trade my health for 10 minutes of pleasure," he says. "To satisfy my hunger on the run, I started to munch on fresh fruits and vegetables."

He also began a "moderate" exercise program. The first day, he tried to run about a mile from the Capitol to the Washington Mon-

ument and nearly coughed up a lung. "So I tried a more sensible approach, walking 20 minutes every day, occasionally revving up the pace to a jog for a few minutes," he says. "After a month, I was running the whole 20 minutes, and I began increasing my time."

Two months later, Salmon had lost 40 pounds, and his once-chronic heartburn and back pain were gone. "I realized that even though I was pushing 40, I wasn't such an old man after all. Then I got this crazy idea to run a marathon," he says. By race day, he'd lost a total of 70 pounds.

BREAKFAST

6 ounces orange juice

½ toasted cinnamon raisin English muffin topped with 2 tablespoons reduced-fat ricotta cheese

LUNCH

Peanut butter and jelly sandwich made with 2 tablespoons peanut butter, ¼ cup jam, and 2 slices whole wheat bread

½ cup carrot-raisin salad

DINNER

1 roasted chicken drumstick

1 baked sweet potato topped with ⅓ cup crushed pineapple packed in juice (Canned fruits are a great way to add flavor and are more nutritious than honey or brown sugar.)

1 cup steamed broccoli topped with 1 ounce shredded Monterey Jack cheese

1 Chocolate Indulgence cake (see page 143)

SNACK

1 cup low-fat fruit yogurt (For more satisfaction, toss in some berries.)

Diabetes Alert

According to the latest research, diet may be the leading risk factor for diabetes—and the most effective treatment.

Diet—what you eat, and in some cases, what you don't—is at the heart of any diabetes treatment program. The following cutting-edge eating plan not only includes lots of fruits, veggies, and whole grains, it also offers the right amounts of key nutrients while allowing you the flexibility to create meals that you find enjoyable.

And here's a great bonus: This plan will help you lose weight because you'll be cutting calories. "Being overweight is clearly your biggest modifiable diabetes risk factor," says Harvard researcher Caren G. Solomon, M.D.

The Eat to Beat Diabetes Diet

This exclusive plan combines the best of the best. It brings you every top nutrition strategy likely to increase your chances of beating diabetes and reaping the joys of good health. And it's also designed to allow you to lose or control weight—another way you can fight diabetes.

Studies show that choosing the foods in this diet should lower your risk not only of diabetes and obesity but also of heart attack, high blood pressure,

stroke, cancer, osteoporosis, and many other chronic illnesses. Start following these 10 steps today, and you'll feel better almost immediately.

Step 1: Eat nine servings of vegetables and fruits every day

Veggies and fruits are the foundation of the Eat to Beat Diabetes Diet—as opposed to grains, the foundation of the traditional Food Guide Pyramid. You'll be eating nine ½-cup servings of

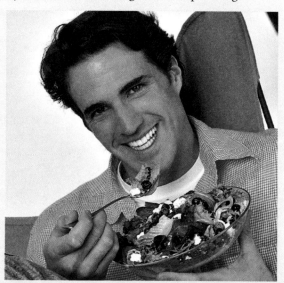

More Is Better

Diets highest in fruits and vegetables are linked to lower risk of diabetes as well as cancer, heart disease, and osteoporosis.

a variety of fruits and veggies a day. Sound like overkill? In reality, it could spell extra life. Study after study links diets highest in fruits and vegetables with a lower incidence of diabetes and other diseases. More and more experts are saying that five a day should be the minimum and that nine a day—five vegetables and four fruits—is the optimum. Yet most Americans get only four a day.

Step 2: Eat three to six whole grain foods every day

Diets high in whole grains are linked to a lower incidence diabetes as well as heart disease, stroke, and cancer. If you've been eating a high-carbohydrate diet with lots of refined grains—typically, breads, rolls, bagels, pretzels, and crackers made from white flour—it may be a challenge at first to find whole grain substitutes.

But the payoff is worth it. To your body, refined white flour is the same as sugar, making a diet high in white-flour foods the same as a high-sugar diet.

Whole grains also mean extra fiber, which is the closest thing to a magic bullet for weight loss. Not only does it fill you up quickly with fewer calories, it also eliminates some of the calories you eat.

Fiber whisks calories through your digestive system so quickly that some of them never have a chance to end up on your hips.

To maximize fiber's slimming powers, aim for 25 to 35 grams a day. By eating 30 grams a day, your body will absorb almost 120 fewer calories a day. That adds up to a 13-pound loss in 1 year!

Step 3: Eat two or three calcium-rich foods every day

Not only does adequate calcium support strong bones and help prevent osteoporosis, but clinical studies suggest that it also helps prevent high blood pressure as well as colon cancer and PMS. Since diabetes is a risk factor for heart disease, you'll want to keep your blood pressure down. Calcium may also lower your body fat, which, in turn, will help your body use insulin more efficiently. A group of women who ate at least 1,000 milligrams of calcium a day, along with a diet of no more than 1,900 calories daily, lost more weight—as much as 6 pounds more—during a 2-year study than women who ate less calcium.

Obvious high-calcium choices include 1% and fat-free milk, low-fat and fat-free yogurt, and reduced-fat and fat-free cheese. Other good choices are orange and grapefruit juices and soy milk that have been fortified with calcium. To equal the calcium found in milk, look for at least 30 percent of the Daily Value (DV) for calcium per serving.

If you are age 50 or older or have low bone density, you should be getting 1,500 milligrams of calcium a day. (If you're younger, aim for 1,000 milligrams a day.)

Step 4: Eat beans at least five times a week

Beans are the highest-fiber foods you can find, with the single exception of breakfast cereals made with wheat bran. Diets high in fiber are linked to

Cut the Salt

To reduce sodium in canned beans by about one-third, rinse off the canning liquid before using. Or look for canned beans with no added sodium.

a lower incidence of diabetes and other chronic diseases such as cancer, heart disease, stroke, and even ulcers. Beans are especially high in soluble fiber, which lowers cholesterol levels, and folate, which lowers levels of another risk factor for heart disease: homocysteine.

Step 5: Nosh on nuts five times a week

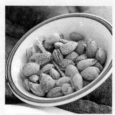

Studies show that people who eat nuts regularly have a lower incidence of heart disease and other illness than people who avoid them. (People with diabetes are at increased risk of heart disease.) Even among the healthiest eaters, the ones who also eat nuts have the best health record. Exactly why isn't known yet, but one reason could be compounds in nuts called to-cotrienols.

Keep a jar of chopped nuts in your fridge. Sprinkle 2 tablespoons a day on cereal, yogurt, veggies, salads, or wherever the crunch and rich flavor appeal to you.

Step 6: Feast on fish

Studies show that people who eat fish twice a week have fewer fatal heart attacks. Scientists credit omega-3 fats, which have the ability to prevent the development of a dangerously irregular heartbeat.

The protein in fish is a great hunger-stopper and, when combined with those naughty carbohydrates, can help keep your blood sugar in check. Protein also helps build healthy muscles that burn tons of calories. "Fish is an excellent source of protein because it's high in omega-3 fatty acids that are good for your heart while low in cholesterol and saturated fat," says Michael Hamilton, M.P.H., M.D., associate professor of research at the Pennington Biomedical Research Center in Baton Rouge, Louisiana. To get the most omega-3s, choose salmon, white albacore tuna canned in water, rainbow trout, anchovies, herring, sardines, and mackerel.

Step 7: Drink at least eight glasses of water every day, plus a cup or more of tea

Every cell in your body needs water to function. Not only does drinking lots of water help you feel full, but people who drink plenty of water also appear to get fewer colon and bladder cancers. A cup of tea provides a strong infusion of antioxidants that help keep blood from clotting too easily (which may thwart heart attacks—important to people with diabetes) and that may help lower your risk of cancer and rheumatoid arthritis.

Step 8: Stick to your fat budget

To stay within a healthy fat budget—25 percent of calories from fat—you must first find the maximum fat allowance for your calorie level. Once you know your fat budget, see whether you're staying within the bounds by adding up the grams of fat for all the food that you eat in a day.

Try to get most of your fat from olive and canola oils (or salad dressings made from them), trans-free margarine, nuts, and fish. And spread

Know Your Fat Budget

Here's how many grams you can eat a day based on the number of calories you consume.

Calories	Fat (g)
1,250	35
1,500	42
1,750	49
2,000	56
2,250	63

your fat throughout the day—just a little helps you absorb fat-soluble nutrients from vegetables and fruit.

Step 9: Take some sensible nutrition insurance

Besides following your fabulous diet, take a multivitamin/mineral supplement. You'll also want to add these individual supplements.

- 100 to 500 milligrams of vitamin C
- 100 to 400 IU of vitamin E
- 500 to 1,000 milligrams of calcium

Step 10: Consider your options carefully

These choices are up to you with the Eat to Beat Diabetes Diet.

Meat and poultry. If you want, you can choose up to 3 cooked ounces (the size of a deck of cards) a day. But you'll get enough protein on the Eat to Beat Diabetes Diet without adding meat, and studies consistently link vegetarian diets to better health, perhaps partly be-

cause diets low in meat are naturally lower in saturated fat.

Eggs. If you have diabetes or high cholesterol or are overweight, you can eat up to four eggs a week.

Alcohol. Whether you can drink alcohol with diabetes largely depends on the medication that you're taking. Check with your doctor for advice on how alcohol may interact with your particular medication.

Sweets. Reserve them for special occasions. Talk to your doctor or a registered dietitian if you'd like to incorporate sweets into your diet. In general, it's a good idea to avoid high-sugar foods, which offer lots of empty calories and not much else.

Servings to Strive For

Use this at-a-glance guide to keep track of your food intake for your Eat to Beat Diabetes Diet.

Servings per Day

- Vegetables and fruits
  . . . . 9 (5 veggie/4 fruit)
- Whole grains. 3–6
- High-calcium foods. 2–3
- Water. . . . 8 or more glasses
- Tea . . . . 1 or more cups

Servings per Week

- Beans . . . . 5 or more
- Nuts 5
- Fish. 2

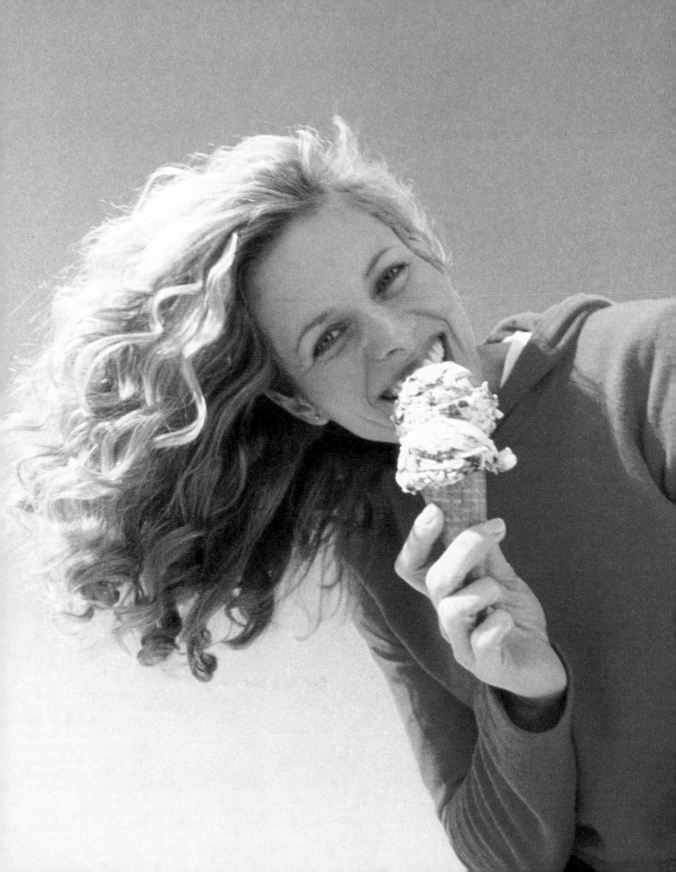

PART SIX

Naughty Foods Gone Good

You'll be surprised how good these once-maligned treats are for your health and your waistline.

CHAPTER 15

Say Hello to Some Old Favorites

Guess what? Pizza, ice cream, and even cheese can be good for you!

Ever feel as if only foods you hate are relegated to the "healthiest foods on the planet?" Ever wish yummy foods would make that list? Well, your wish has finally come true. Science has rescued some of our "naughtiest" foods from the taboo list. New studies have identified a number of former no-nos that actually add to better health and longer life. In effect, some of our vices have turned into virtues!

Think chocolate and nuts and cooking oil. Think pizza. Think ice cream. They have all made the "healthy list." Steady, now. You can't go hog-wild with Dove bars, Brie, and supersize burgers, or you'll overdose on calories and saturated fat. That's an invitation to obesity, clogged arteries, cancer, and diabetes. But enjoying just enough of the following six once-forbidden treats may actually boost your diet's health quotient.

‖ Pizza

Pizza sauce delivers tons of lycopene, a carotenoid found at high levels in the blood and prostates of men with lower rates of prostate cancer. And the cheese provides calcium, which helps build bone, lower blood pressure, and inhibit colon cancer.

Because a 12-inch double sausage and pepperoni pizza delivers more than 2,000 calories and 60 grams of saturated fat, you should hold yourself to two slices of thin-crust veggie pizza, which weigh in at just 300 calories and 2.5 grams of saturated fat.

Patronize shops that pile on the sauce and veggies but just lightly oil the pan. (Place your slice on a napkin to detect pizza with a greasy bottom.) Gotta have meat? Add it at home by precooking pepperoni or sausage then blotting the grease on paper towels before adding the meat to the pizza. Or you could use low-fat Canadian bacon, then season with anise seed or hot peppers to mimic sausage.

‖ Ice Cream

As long as you choose the right ice cream, you'll get a very impressive dose of calcium for your bones and your blood pressure. Look for a variety with 15 percent of the Daily Value (DV) for calcium in every ½-cup serving. That way, a double portion (1 cup) gives you as much calcium as an 8-ounce glass of milk—300 milligrams.

Officially, one serving of ice cream is ½ cup— the size of a tennis ball. Stick to this amount if you're eating calorie- and fat-loaded premium ice cream (one with 250 calories or more per ½ cup).

I DID IT!

Sandra Hameroff: Pizza and French Fries Helped Her Lose Postpregnancy Pounds

Shortly after the birth of her son, Noah, Sandra Hameroff was determined to return to her prepregnancy weight of 100 pounds. She went on a strict diet, denying herself many of her favorite foods. She found herself on the brink of a full-scale binge more than once.

When a sympathetic friend learned of Hameroff's efforts—and her list of forbidden foods—she made a suggestion: "Why not give yourself a break from your eating program once a week? You'll tame those cravings before they permanently undo your diet."

The next Monday through Thursday, Hameroff was a model of gastronomic self-control, amazing even herself. Then came Friday, and with it, her old favorites: pizza and a hearty dessert.

The next day, she resumed her stricter eating plan with greater enthusiasm. Soon after, her husband got into the act by taking her to dinner on Friday nights, which only served to make her splurges seem even more special. "I looked forward to them," she says. "They made my diet easier to stick with."

Four months later, Hameroff stepped on a scale and discovered that she had lost all 40 pounds without guilt or giving up the foods that she loved.

But if you're eating regular or low-fat brands, 1 cup is fine.

If you can't keep a "high-vulnerability" half-gallon on hand, go to an ice cream shop and buy just one scoop. At home, have an ice cream on a stick, or buy just enough so that everyone in your family gets one scoop. Consulting nutritionist Robyn Flipse, R.D., recommends serving ice cream in a stemmed 6-ounce wine glass. "It looks elegant—and you must stop with a small amount," she says.

Chocolate

Chocolate, especially the dark or bittersweet kind, is rich in flavonoids, antioxidants that protect your heart by preventing platelets from sticking together and forming clots that could cause a heart attack. But even milk chocolate is good: A typical 1½-ounce bar packs as much antioxidant power as a 5-ounce glass of red wine.

Unfortunately, too much chocolate winds up on your hips. That same 1½-ounce chocolate bar loads on 234 calories. That's more than 10 percent of the calories that most women need for a whole day. If you crave a daily dose of chocolate, stick with about 100 calories' worth. That's about four Hershey's Kisses. Try individually wrapped mini or fun-size chocolate bars such as Nestlé Crunch or plain chocolate. At 50 calories each, you can have two.

natural WONDER

OMEGASMART CHEESE
Canadian farmers have created a heart-smart cheese by feeding their cows a fish-meal formula. The result is OmegaSmart cheese, with 112 milligrams of omega-3 fatty acids per 1-ounce serving.

Cheese

The news about cheese—except the fat-free kind—is that it contains a special kind of fat called conjugated linoleic acid, or CLA, that scientists are investigating as a new weapon against breast cancer. And all that concentrated calcium—300 milligrams, as much as a glass of milk, in just 1½ ounces of Cheddar—is a boon for bone health. And finally, there's your smile: Eating hard cheese at the end of a meal can protect your pearly whites from tooth decay.

Of course, cheese contains cholesterol-raising saturated fat: 1½ ounces of Cheddar packs 9 grams. For most women, that's more than half of the saturated fat that you should have in a day. Hold yourself to 1½ ounces, the size of about six dice. If you're eating strong-flavored cheese, such as extra-sharp Cheddar or Gorgonzola, you'll be satisfied with less.

Nuts

Several large studies have linked nuts to lower heart disease risk and longer life. In the landmark Nurses' Health Study, for instance, women who ate the most nuts (about 5 ounces per week) had half the risk of heart attack as those who rarely ate them. Although the power source in nuts is unclear, researchers suggest that their unsaturated fats, magnesium, copper, folate, protein, potassium, fiber, and vitamin E may all play a part.

Nuts are a high-calorie treat, weighing in at about 180 calories per ounce (that's about a scant

Don't Char That Steak

In a dramatic study, women who ate hamburger, steak, and bacon very well done were more than 4½ times as likely to get breast cancer as women who ate these meats cooked rare or medium.

How come? Could be nasty compounds called heterocyclic amines (HAs) that form in meat when it's cooked beyond the just-done stage, says Mark Knize, HA project leader at Lawrence Livermore National Lab in Livermore, California. In animals, HAs are known to cause cancer.

For meat with the least HAs, follow these tips.

Roast, steam, or stew. Oven roasting makes it easier to control temperature and avoid overcooking. Steaming or stewing keeps meat moist, which inhibits the formation of HAs.

Avoid grilling, broiling, or frying until the charred stage. When the meat dries out, more HAs can form.

If you must grill, marinate first. If you marinate chicken before you grill it, the levels of HAs drop dramatically.

Don't undercook. Do cook meat beyond the rare or medium-rare stage to just done to make sure you kill illness-causing bacteria.

¼ cup). Several studies suggest that eating a handful (about an ounce) of nuts two to five times a week gets the job done without packing on the pounds.

‖ Beef

Beef is one of the richest and best-absorbed sources of zinc, a key mineral in your immune system's fight against many enemies, from viruses to cancer. Getting enough zinc is also critical for appetite, taste, and night vision, yet only half of adults over 50 come close to the DV of 15 milligrams.

But plate-size portions of fatty meats such as hamburger and prime rib are loaded with saturated fat, which raises cholesterol and heart dis-

ease risk. A restaurant-size 14-ounce sirloin steak has 27 grams of saturated fat—nearly twice the saturated fat that women should have in a day.

When it comes to beef, portion size is everything. A 3-ounce portion, about the size of a computer mouse or a bath-size bar of soap, is about right, says Flipse. A 3-ounce sirloin steak has 6 grams of saturated fat, 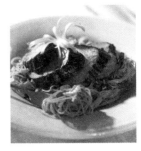 well within a woman's saturated fat maximum of 14 grams.

Choose the "select" grade and stick with lean cuts such as round (top, bottom, eye) and loin (sirloin, tenderloin). Use small portions as flavor enhancers for stir-fries.

CHAPTER 16

The Big Fat Comeback

After years as a nutritional scourge, fat is back—but you must eat the right kinds.

Here's a shocker. Turns out, fat is so good for you that you probably should be eating more of it.

Specifically, you need more smart fats: omega-3 fats (from foods such as salmon and walnuts) and monounsaturated fats (from delicacies such as olive oil, almonds, and avocados). Research shows that people who eat more of these fats have a lower incidence of cancer, heart disease, depression, asthma, even Alzheimer's disease. Smart fats can help control diabetes and high blood pressure, too.

Make no mistake though: Too much total fat—more than 25 percent of calories—is still a bad idea. You want to limit saturated fats and trans fats, and curb the omega-6 fats, such as corn oil.

Try these easy tips to get the right balance of smart fats in your diet.

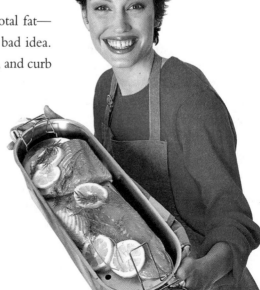

Eating More Omega-3s

There are two main omega-3 sources: fish, which provides eicosapentaenoic acid (EPA) and docosahexaenoic acid (DHA); and plants, which have alpha-linolenic acid (ALA). Foods with high EPA and DHA include salmon, mackerel, sardines, herring, anchovies, rainbow trout, bluefish, caviar, and white albacore tuna. Foods with ALA include canola oil, flaxseed, flaxseed oil, walnuts, walnut oil, and dark green leafy vegetables.

Omega-3 expert Penny Kris-Etherton, R.D., Ph.D., distinguished professor of nutrition at Pennsylvania State University in University Park, recommends at least 0.5 gram of EPA and DHA per day. For ALA, she recommends about 1 gram per day minimum.

Here are eight ways to boost your omega-3 consumption from fish, flax, and other foods.

1. Eat fatty fish twice a week. That way, you'll average about 0.5 gram of EPA and DHA per day.
2. Make tuna salad sandwiches. Buy canned white albacore tuna in water (light tuna has less omega-3). A 3-ounce serving of tuna averages 1.1 grams of DHA and EPA. (Restaurant tuna is mostly yellowfin, not a high-omega-3 fish.)
3. Order pizza with anchovies. Five anchovies have 0.4 gram of EPA and DHA.
4. Make a mini-meal of sardines with whole wheat toast. Two sardines have 0.36 gram of DHA and EPA.
5. Celebrate with caviar. One tablespoon has 1 gram of omega-3s.

Store Good Fat in Your Seat

When scientists want to find out what fats are actually consumed, just asking people is notoriously unreliable. To be certain, you need to take a sample of fat from the buttocks and analyze it.

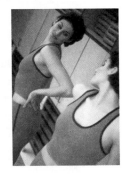

And when 200 people—half of them heart attack survivors—submitted to such a test, the results showed what a dramatic difference the right or wrong fats can make. The people with the most healthy omega-3 fat from fish stored in their buttocks had only one-fifth the risk of heart attack. People with the most cholesterol-raising trans fat had more than double the risk of heart attack.

6. Use canola oil for baking and cooking. Buy mayonnaise, margarine, and salad dressing made with canola oil. One tablespoon of canola oil has 1.3 grams of ALA.
7. Make salad dressing from walnut oil and red wine vinegar. One tablespoon of walnut oil has 1.4 grams of ALA.
8. Sprinkle ground flaxseed on cereal or yogurt. One tablespoon of flaxseed has 2.2 grams of ALA. You can buy flaxseed at health food stores or natural food supermarkets such as Fresh Fields.

Buy the Fattiest Tuna

Choose cans of water-packed white tuna with the highest fat content. Fat can range from 0.5 to 5 grams per serving. The more total fat, the more omega-3s.

Eating More Monounsaturates

You'll find monos in olive oil, olives, canola oil (also a good source of omega-3s), most nuts (almonds, cashews, pecans, pistachios), avocados, peanuts, and peanut butter. Up to 15 percent or more of daily calories should come from these sources.

Here are seven ways to get more monounsaturates.

1. Buy salad dressing made with olive oil or make your own. (Bonus: A dressing with fat means that you absorb more protective carotenoids from your veggies.)

2. Sprinkle 1 tablespoon of toasted, chopped nuts a day on cereal, yogurt, stir-fries, casseroles, rice dishes, or cream soups.

3. Dip crusty bread in olive oil.

4. Opt for olive oil in cooking. Though you can find special high-mono sunflower and safflower oils (called high-oleic), they're not good substitutes for olive oil since they lack the disease-fighting phytochemicals that olive oil contains.

5. Savor peanut butter—in moderate amounts (1 to 2 tablespoons).

6. Appreciate avocados. Stop passing up this delicious treat. One quarter of an avocado packs 4.5 grams of monounsaturates.

7. Flavor up with olives. Add punch to salads and casseroles with chopped olives.

Keeping Omega-6 Fats in Check

Omega-6 fats in vegetable oils such as corn oil are essential; our diets must have some of these polyunsaturated fats. But we've gone overboard and need to cut back.

Experts think humans evolved on a diet of equal portions of omega-6 and omega-3 fats. Today, because we eat so much corn and soybean oils, we get 10 to 20 times more omega-6s than the Stone Age person. In your body, that hinders the work of omega-3s. It lowers LDL cholesterol but also can reduce healthy HDL cholesterol. Some research hints that it could also encourage breast cancer.

Omega-6-rich foods include vegetable oils made from corn, cottonseed, safflower seed, sun-

Pick the Right Salmon

Most salmon, including the farm-raised kind, is rich in omega-3s. The exceptions are smoked salmon and lox. During processing, they lose most of their fat, including omega-3s.

Smart Switches

All fats are high in calories—9 calories per gram. To avoid gaining weight when you add smart fats to your diet, use them to replace a fat that's not so good for you.

Instead Of . . .	Choose . . .	Smart Fat Payoff
3 oz broiled sirloin (229 calories, 14.2 g fat)	3 oz roasted Atlantic farmed salmon (175 calories, 10.5 g fat)	+ 1.8 g omega-3 fats (DHA and EPA) − 3.5 g saturated fat
Topping salad with ¼ c shredded Cheddar cheese (114 calories, 9.3 g fat)	1.5 Tbsp chopped toasted almonds (125 calories, 11 g fat)	+ 4.5 g monounsaturated fat − 4.9 g saturated fat
Sautéing in 2 tsp corn oil (80 calories, 9.1 g fat)	2 tsp canola oil (83 calories, 9.4 g fat)	+ 3.3 g monounsaturated fat + 0.8 g omega-3 fats (ALA) − 3.4 g omega-6 fat
Topping pizza wedge with 11 pepperoni slices (55 calories, 4.8 g fat)	5 anchovies (42 calories, 1.9 g fat)	+ 0.4 g omega-3 fats (DHA and EPA)
Spreading bread with 2 tsp butter (68 calories, 7.7 g fat)	2 tsp olive oil (80 calories, 9 g fat)	+ 4.4 g monounsaturated fat − 3.6 g saturated fat

flower seed, and soybeans. (Soybean oil has more healthy omega-3s than many oils, but it also has very high levels of omega-6s.)

Aim for no more than four times as much omega-6s as you get of omega-3s, or about 6 grams a day. Don't worry if that sounds complicated—our tips make it happen easily.

Here are three ways to tame your omega-6 intake.

1. Margarine and mayonnaise are often made from soybean or other high omega-6 oils. Look for brands made from canola oil.
2. Make or buy salad dressing with olive oil. Bottled salad dressings are often soybean-oil based.
3. Use olive or canola oil for cooking or baking instead of corn, safflower, or sunflower oils.

CHAPTER 17

Spread the Word about Peanut Butter

America's favorite condiment is good for your heart—and your waistline.

Here's great news: Recent research now proves that peanut butter is actually very, very good for you. Its healthy monounsaturated fat—eaten as the main fat in a sensible diet—can lower your risks for heart disease and diabetes, and even help you lose weight!

Skeptical? In one study, researchers divided 101 overweight people into two groups. One group limited fat to a very low 20 percent of calories. The other group ate mo-nounsaturated-fat foods such as peanut butter, which boosted their fat total to a rich 35 percent of calories.

The results? Both groups lost about 11 pounds in the first 6 weeks. But twice as many peanut butter dieters stuck it out, and they maintained their weight for 18 months. Why? Taste, first and foremost. People have to enjoy what they eat to stick with it.

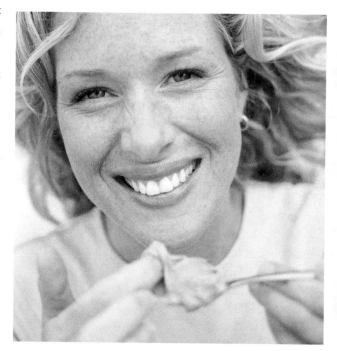

The Peanut Butter Diet

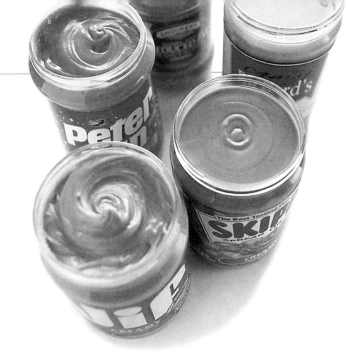

Peanut butter is so good for you that *Prevention* magazine recently created the Peanut Butter Diet, an easy 5-day eating plan that lets you indulge in 4 to 6 tablespoons of peanut butter every day—guilt-free!

On the diet, a satisfying 30 to 35 percent of calories come from fat, mostly monounsaturated fat from peanut butter. Yet the plan holds the line at 1,500 nutrition-packed calories for women and 2,200 for men. This means that you'll drop about ½ pound a week—or 25 pounds in a year! Men, to boost your calories to about 2,200, double each food marked with ★★, and triple each food marked with ★★★.

Monday

BREAKFAST

PB Oatmeal: Stir up ¼ cup dry old-fashioned oats, 1 cup fat-free milk, and 4 dried apricot halves, cut into quarters. Microwave for 3 minutes, then stir in 2 tablespoons chunky peanut butter and ¼ teaspoon ground cinnamon.

LUNCH

2 cups mixed salad greens, ½ cup canned kidney beans★★ (rinsed and drained), and a small chopped pear tossed with 2 teaspoons extra-virgin olive oil, 2 teaspoons balsamic vinegar, ¼ teaspoon dried basil, and a sprinkle of garlic powder

1 slice multigrain bread★★★

SNACK

¾ cup tomato juice

DINNER

2 ounces lean pork tenderloin and ½ cup each snow peas, broccoli florets, and slivered red bell peppers stir-fried in 1 teaspoon peanut oil. Season with 1 tablespoon low-sodium soy sauce and 1 teaspoon Asian five-spice powder. Serve over ½ cup cooked brown rice.★★★

TREAT

PB Pudding: In a microwaveable dessert dish, microwave 2 tablespoons peanut butter until melted, about 1 minute. Quickly stir in ¾ cup fat-free plain yogurt. Top with a small sliced banana.

Day's Total: *1,500 calories, 76 g protein, 199 g carbohydrates, 55 g fat, 10 g saturated fat, 26 g monounsaturated fat, 37 g dietary fiber, 1,993 mg sodium, 808 mg calcium*

Tuesday

BREAKFAST

1 cup Multi-Bran Chex★★ with ½ cup frozen wild blueberries and 1 cup fat-free milk

LUNCH

1 cup salad greens, ¼ cup shredded carrots, ¼ cup shredded red cabbage, ⅛ avocado cut in chunks, and 1 tablespoon chopped hazelnuts tossed with 1 teaspoon extra-virgin olive oil and 2 teaspoons balsamic vinegar. Stuff into a small whole wheat pita pocket.

1 cup fat-free plain yogurt

SNACK

PB Apple: Slice a red Delicious apple and spread with 2 tablespoons peanut butter.

DINNER

2 ounces thinly sliced lean eye of round beef,★★★ 1 small sliced yellow onion, 1 large sliced portobello mushroom, and 1 minced clove garlic sautéed in 1 teaspoon olive oil

5 steamed frozen asparagus spears

1 small baked sweet potato★★ dusted with pumpkin pie spice

QUICK & HEALTHY

CREAMY GINGERED CARROT SOUP

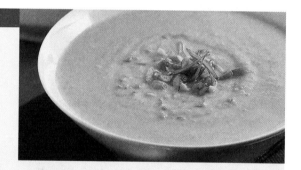

Here's a carrot soup made velvety from potatoes and milk and made more flavorful by peanut butter.

1	tablespoon peanut oil
1	pound baby carrots
2	ribs celery, chopped
1	large white or yellow onion, sliced
4½	cups water
2	cups fat-free milk
1	pound baking potatoes, peeled and sliced (about 2 large potatoes)
⅓	cup creamy peanut butter (with salt)
2	tablespoons minced fresh ginger (or 2 teaspoons ground ginger)
1½	teaspoons salt
1½	teaspoons white pepper

Place a stockpot over low heat. Add the oil, carrots, celery, and onion, then cover. Stir occasionally for 8 minutes, or until the onions are translucent.

Add the water, milk, potatoes, peanut butter, ginger, salt, and pepper. Cover and bring to a boil. Reduce the heat. Simmer, uncovered, until the veggies are tender, about 25 minutes.

In a blender, puree the soup in batches. Return the pureed soup to the clean stockpot. Adjust the seasonings. Heat through over low heat.

MAKES 6 SERVINGS

Per serving: 232 calories, 9 g protein, 30 g carbohydrates, 10 g fat, 2 g saturated fat, 5 g monounsaturated fat, 1 mg cholesterol, 5 g dietary fiber, 732 mg sodium

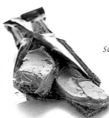

TREAT

PB Granola Bar: Spread a fat-free date-almond granola bar★★ with 2 tablespoons peanut butter.★★

Day's Total: *1,535 calories, 73 g protein, 218 g carbohydrates, 55 g fat, 11 g saturated fat, 28 g monounsaturated fat, 34 g dietary fiber, 1,493 mg sodium, 890 mg calcium*

Wednesday

BREAKFAST

PB Shake: In a blender, whip together 1 cup fat-free milk, 1 small ripe banana, 2 tablespoons toasted wheat germ,★★ and 2 tablespoons peanut butter.

LUNCH

1 cup instant black bean soup
½ cup raw broccoli florets
½ cup grapes

SNACK

1 cup calcium-fortified orange juice

DINNER

3 ounces broiled salmon★★
½ cup cooked whole wheat couscous★★★
1 cup brussels sprouts
1 cup yellow squash cooked in 3 teaspoons olive oil

TREAT

PB Toast: Toast 1 slice whole wheat bread★★★ and spread with 2 tablespoons peanut butter.★★

Day's Total: *1,536 calories, 78 g protein, 195 g carbohydrates, 60 g fat, 11 g saturated fat, 28 g monoun-*

saturated fat, 36 g dietary fiber, 1,708 mg sodium, 988 mg calcium

Thursday

BREAKFAST

1 egg (or ¼ cup egg substitute) scrambled with ¼ cup each chopped green bell pepper and onion (frozen is fine) in 1 teaspoon canola oil. Season with salt and pepper.
2 clementines
1 slice whole wheat bread★★★

LUNCH

Open-faced tomato melt made by topping 1 slice whole wheat bread★★ with 1 thick slice fresh tomato★★ and 1 slice reduced-fat Cheddar cheese,★★ then broiling in a toaster oven until cheese melts
1 medium banana

SNACK

PB Celery: Stuff a large celery rib★★ with 2 tablespoons peanut butter.★★

DINNER

1 cup dry whole wheat macaroni,★★ cooked then topped with 1 cup low-fat mushroom-and-pepper pasta sauce. Add 12 large steamed shrimp★★ and 2 tablespoons grated Parmesan cheese.
2 cups salad greens tossed with 2 teaspoons extra-virgin olive oil and 1 tablespoon balsamic vinegar

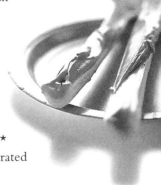

QUICK & HEALTHY

CHINESE CHICKEN SALAD WITH PEANUT BUTTER DRESSING

Once you try this Asian-inspired salad, it will become a mainstay of your meal repertoire. It's also a great way to use leftover grilled or baked chicken breasts.

Peanut Butter Dressing

2	teaspoons peanut oil
2	teaspoons toasted sesame oil
¼	cup creamy peanut butter (with salt)
¼	cup rice vinegar
	Juice of 1 lime
1½	tablespoons soy sauce
1	tablespoon honey
1	clove garlic
1	tablespoon chunk fresh ginger (or 1 teaspoon ground ginger)
1	teaspoon chili powder

Chinese Chicken Salad

4	small (approximately 14 ounces total) grilled or baked boneless, skinless chicken breast halves, sliced into long, bite-size pieces
8	cups mesclun or other mixed lettuce greens
¼	cup chopped fresh cilantro

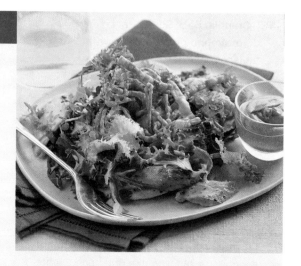

To make the dressing: In a blender or food processor, puree the oils, peanut butter, vinegar, lime juice, soy sauce, honey, garlic, ginger, and chili powder.

To make the salad: Mix the chicken, greens, and cilantro. Just before serving, toss the salad with the dressing. Garnish as desired.

MAKES 4 SERVINGS

Per serving: 348 calories, 37 g protein, 15 g carbohydrates, 16 g fat, 3 g saturated fat, 7 g monounsaturated fat, 83 mg cholesterol, 4 g dietary fiber, 628 mg sodium

TREAT

PB Dates: Fill 4 large dates with 2 tablespoons peanut butter.

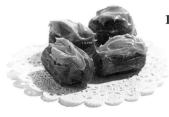

Day's Total: *1,495 calories, 72 g protein, 183 g carbohydrates, 62 g fat, 14 g saturated fat, 29 g monounsaturated fat, 30 g dietary fiber, 1,947 mg sodium, 661 mg calcium*

Friday

BREAKFAST

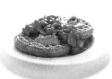

PB Waffles: Toast 2 whole grain waffles,★★ then spread with 2 tablespoons peanut butter.★★ Top with ½ cup thawed, mashed frozen strawberries.

LUNCH

2 cups baby spinach, ¼ cup sliced red onion, 5 grape tomatoes, and 2 ounces flaked white water-packed tuna★★ tossed with 1 teaspoon extra-virgin olive oil and 2 teaspoon red wine vinegar. Season with freshly ground black pepper and ¼ teaspoon dried oregano

1 navel orange

SNACK

2 cinnamon graham crackers★★★

1 kiwifruit

DINNER

½ cup sliced yellow onion and 2 ounces diced chicken breast★★ sautéed in 2 teaspoons olive oil. Stir into 1 cup cooked wild rice.★★ Top with ½ tablespoon toasted chopped pecans.

1 cup cooked carrots

TREAT

PB Sundae: Microwave 2 tablespoons peanut butter for about 1 minute (until melted). Drizzle over ½ cup Edy's or Dreyer's fat-free frozen yogurt.

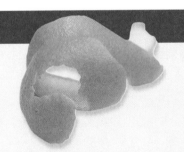

Day's Total: *1,534 calories, 72 g protein, 184 g carbohydrates, 61 g fat, 11 g saturated fat, 28 g monounsaturated fat, 29 g dietary fiber, 1,230 mg sodium, 698 mg calcium*

QUICK & HEALTHY

TROPICAL PEANUT BUTTER DIPPING SAUCE

A quick-to-fix dip packed with phytochemicals and fruity flavor. This is a great dip for raw vegetables or cut fruit.

¼	**cup creamy peanut butter (with salt)**
¼	**cup apricot fruit spread**
¼	**cup papaya or other tropical fruit juice**
¼	**teaspoon orange peel**
	Fresh cilantro

Mix the peanut butter, fruit spread, fruit juice, and orange peel in a saucepan.

Place over medium-high heat, stirring until the mixture just starts to bubble.

Remove from the heat. Serve warm with a fresh cilantro garnish.

MAKES 4 SERVINGS

Per serving: 154 calories, 4 g protein, 19 g carbohydrates, 8 g fat, 2 g saturated fat, 4 g monounsaturated fat, 0 mg cholesterol, 1 g dietary fiber, 82 mg sodium

CHAPTER 18

Great News for Chocoholics

Discover why you can and should eat this decadent treat every day.

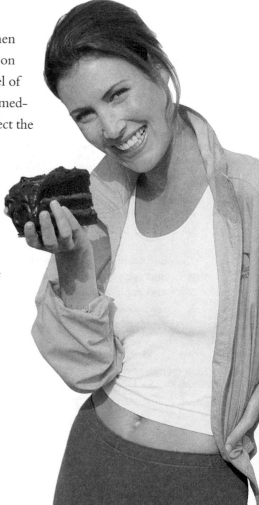

It may be the last thing that crosses your mind when you bite into that milky, sweet piece of heaven here on earth called chocolate. But each time you let a morsel of it melt in your mouth, you're taking a dose of herbal medicine packed with a wild array of compounds that affect the brain and nervous system.

Chocolate is derived from the cacao (cocoa) bean, which has been used for its medicinal powers throughout history. People in modern Latin America still rely on the cacao bean as a mind tonic. Are they on to something? Definitely.

As it turns out, special compounds in chocolate can improve your mood, fire up your energy, reduce your appetite, and even spark some romance. Here's how it works.

Natural Mood Booster

A USDA survey found that Americans consume more chocolate in the notoriously blue winter months than in any other season. Another study of 853 female university students revealed that they ate more chocolate when they had premenstrual tension.

Cacao beans contain a variety of amino acids

Chocolate Tonic

Planet Botanic, an herbal research group in London, uses a beverage made from cacao beans to treat mild depression, exhaustion, and poor sex drive. This special tonic also works in weight-loss plans and to wean people off chocolate-bar addiction.

Here's how to make this concoction in your own kitchen.

1. Take 24 raw cacao beans (you can buy them in Latin American grocery stores) and place them in a pan on the stove. Heat them on low, stirring constantly, for 5 minutes, and then take them out of the pan to cool.

2. Once cool, grind the beans to a fine powder using an electric coffee grinder.

3. Add the powder to 3½ cups of boiling water and boil for 5 minutes. Remove from the heat.

4. While cooling, sweeten to taste. Any sweetener you enjoy is fine.

The result—3 cups of genuine cacao. You can drink it hot or cold. Store in the refrigerator for no more than a week.

Note: If you cannot find the beans, buy organic cacao powder from your health food store. Three teaspoonfuls boiled in 3 cups of water makes the equivalent of the recipe above made from the beans.

How to Use This Chocolate Tonic

For an energy boost: Drink 1 cup three times a day.

To curb your appetite: Drink 1 cup three times a day.

To rev up romance: Drink 1½ cups half an hour before sex.

To wean yourself off chocolate bars: Have 1 cup when the urge hits (maximum 3 cups a day).

Note: Though cacao beans are considered to be safe, they're not recommended for pregnant and nursing women, anyone with kidney stones, those with acid reflux problems, and migraine sufferers.

known for their mood-boosting abilities, including tryptophan, phenylalanine, and tyrosine. Looking at just one of these amino acids is telling: Tryptophan increases the production of serotonin, which is your body's natural "happy" chemical. The more serotonin your body produces, the happier you feel.

Energy in Every Bite

An interesting combination of the stimulants theobromine, theophylline, and a bit of caffeine gives chocolate its gentle kick-start effect. In one study that looked at the effects of chocolate on the recovery time of recreational runners, those who ate a chocolate bar before running had more energy to spare afterward than those who hadn't eaten chocolate.

While chocolate may provide you with a much-needed energy boost, it probably won't give you the jitters that other stimulants such as highly caffeinated coffee and cola can cause. Why? Because nature balances out the cacao bean's stimulant activity with some natural calming chemicals: valeric acid, a relaxant, and glutamic acid, which reduces anxiety.

Alter Your Appetite

Could your wildest fantasy be true? Could chocolate help you lose weight?

Well . . . maybe. Research has found that the stimulant theobromine suppresses your appetite. In addition, chocolate's long list of feel-good compounds might counteract that bad mood you often find yourself in when trying to lose weight. So chocolate could aid your weight-loss attempts by acting as an appetite suppressant and mood enhancer all in one.

But—and there's a big but—the chocolate most of us eat is rich in animal fat, sugar, and artificial flavoring and has more calories per square inch than most foods on the planet.

If, on the other hand, you use the drink made from cacao beans (see "Chocolate Tonic" on page 167), chocolate may indeed help you drop pounds.

Rev Up for Romance

What does a suitor bring a date? A box of chocolates. Why? Because the chemicals in chocolate seem to get love flowing.

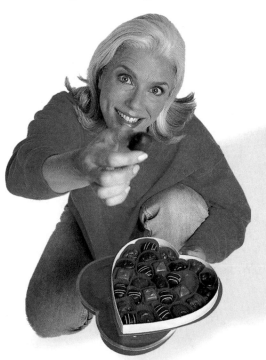

⌐ I DID IT!

Vicki Rogers Givens: She's 70 Pounds Slimmer— And Still Eating Chocolate

Vicki Rogers Givens adores chocolate. She craves chocolate. She eats chocolate. And she still has taken off 70 pounds in 1 year.

She's done it by being choosy about her chocolate treats. Ever since she was a child, Givens, an administrative assistant from Indianapolis, has fought the battle of the bulge. In college, she reached 225 pounds, the most she has ever weighed.

These days, at age 42, Givens is a fit 155 pounds. She says that she reached her goal weight by making smart food substitutions that save calories and still satisfy. "Instead of high-fat chocolate chip cookies, I eat a handful of chocolate animal crackers," she says. They do the trick with far fewer calories and fat. Other favorites include fat-free chocolate pudding, Fudge-sicles, and hot chocolate.

Of all chocolate's facets, this is the least understood. What we do know is that chocolate contains valeric acid, a sedative and tranquilizer. It also has a natural mood booster—the neurotransmitter dopamine. Add to that chocolate's other mood-enhancing qualities, and you have all the ingredients for a relaxed, happy state of mind—the ideal emotional setup for romance.

But there's more to chocolate's aphrodisiac effects. Chocolate contains phytosterols, plant substances that may mimic human sex hormones. Several studies have shown that women crave chocolate just before menstruation, at the moment when hormone levels are at their lowest. Perhaps chocolate provides a hormone blast just when you need it.

CHAPTER 19

Minding Your Peas and Cucumbers

Add butter, sugar, and salt to your veggies— and live longer!

Adam Drewnowski, Ph.D., heads the nutritional sciences program at the University of Washington in Seattle. His research has revealed that many of the disease-fighting compounds in vegetables taste, well, not so hot if we eat them plain. No wonder only about 25 percent of Americans eat even the minimum five servings of fruits and vegetables a day as suggested by the USDA's Food Guide Pyramid.

Dr. Drewnowski's solution to this? Use butter, olive oil, sugar, and salt to mask and mellow those bitter phytochemical flavors. The recipes that follow will show you how.

Can you go overboard, getting too many calories and more fat than is healthy? Dr. Drewnowski says no, as long as you make veggies the main focus of your meal.

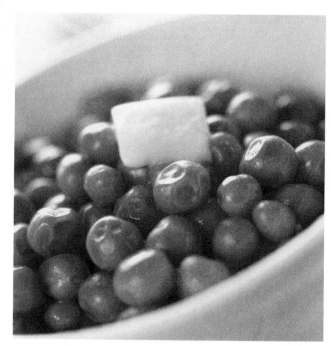

Layered Broccoli Salad
FIGHTS BREAST CANCER

Bring back this favorite recipe that used to be served at many a family picnic and baby shower. Our makeover version saves lots of calories and fat without sacrificing oomph.

Salad

- 6 cups chopped broccoli (cut into ½" bite-size pieces)
- 1 small red onion, very thinly sliced
- 2 ounces shredded extra-sharp Cheddar cheese
- ⅔ cup seedless raisins
- 1½ ounces (about ⅓ cup) dry-roasted peanuts
- 6 slices bacon, cooked and crumbled

Dressing

- 2 tablespoons mayonnaise
- ½ cup fat-free plain yogurt
- ¼ cup sugar
- 1 tablespoon + 2 teaspoons red wine vinegar

In a large glass serving bowl, layer the broccoli, onion, cheese, raisins, and peanuts.

Whisk together the mayonnaise, yogurt, sugar, and vinegar in a bowl or shaker container. Pour the dressing evenly over the salad.

Cover, and refrigerate until ready to serve. Toss on the bacon just before serving.

Makes 6 servings

Per serving: 272 calories, 14 g fat, 3 g dietary fiber

Variation: Use sunflower seeds or chopped, toasted walnuts instead of peanuts.

Sweet Potato Casserole
PROTECTS YOUR HEART

Savor our slimmed-down version of this all-time classic. It is good enough to be served as a super-healthy dessert.

Casserole Filling

- 3 cups cooked, mashed sweet potatoes, without skin (see note)
- ½ cup sugar
- 2 eggs
- 2 teaspoons vanilla extract
- ½ cup fat-free evaporated milk
- 2 tablespoons trans-free margarine, melted

Topping

- ½ cup packed brown sugar
- 1 ounce chopped pecans (about 16 pecan halves)
- ⅓ cup all-purpose flour
- 2 tablespoons butter, melted

Preheat the oven to 350°F. In a large bowl with an electric mixer, blend the potatoes, sugar, eggs, vanilla extract, milk, and margarine. Coat a 13" × 9" baking pan with cooking spray and spread the mixture into the pan.

In a small bowl, combine the sugar, pecans, flour, and butter. Mix very well. Sprinkle the topping mixture evenly over the casserole. (The casserole can be covered and refrigerated for up to 2 days prior to baking.) Bake for 35 to 40 minutes.

Makes 6 servings

Per serving: 410 calories, 13 g fat, 3 g dietary fiber

Note: To save time, use a 40-ounce can of sweet potatoes in light syrup, drained and mashed.

Old-Fashioned Glazed Carrots

FIGHTS BREAST CANCER

Allow a little butter and brown sugar to make cancer-fighting carrots taste just as good as apple pie.

1	**pound baby carrots**
½	**cup water**
2	**tablespoons butter**
4	**teaspoons brown sugar**
	Mint or parsley

In a saucepan, cover and simmer the carrots, water, butter, and brown sugar until the carrots are tender and a syrupy glaze forms on the bottom of the pan. Roll the carrots to coat well with the glaze. Serve with mint or parsley.

Makes 4 servings

Per serving: 72 calories, 6 g fat, 3 g dietary fiber

Sautéed Escarole with Pine Nuts and Raisins

WARDS OFF STROKE

This special green tastes delicious when accompanied by pine nuts and raisins.

1	**tablespoon olive oil**
1	**tablespoon garlic**
¼	**cup pine nuts**
2	**cups cooked escarole**
½	**cup golden raisins**
½	**teaspoon salt**
⅛	**teaspoon ground black pepper**

Heat the olive oil in a 12" skillet over medium heat. Add the garlic and pine nuts and sauté for 1 to 2 minutes, until golden. Add the escarole, raisins, salt, and pepper. Heat through.

Makes 4 servings

Per serving: 177 calories, 9 g fat, 4 g dietary fiber

Mac and Cheese Broccoli

STOPS COLON CANCER

All you need to disguise the bitterness of broccoli is a little cheese.

1	**pound cooked, hot broccoli florets**
	Single serving Stouffer's Macaroni and Cheese Dinner, just cooked and hot

Toss the broccoli with the macaroni and cheese in a serving bowl.

Makes 4 servings

Per serving: 244 calories, 12 g fat, 4 g dietary fiber

⌐ **I DID IT!**

Meredith Willson: Planting a Garden Helped Her Eat More Veggies

A New Year's Eve party to welcome 1994 served as the wake-up call that Meredith Willson needed to get serious about slimming down.

"At the time, I weighed more than 300 pounds," recalls the 43-year-old Athens, Tennessee, resident. "Someone that I hadn't seen in years came up to me and said, 'What happened to the Meredith I used to know?' It was a shock—and shock therapy is a good way to get inspired."

The next day, Willson set her sights on a rather lofty resolution: to lose 120 pounds in 12 months. To do so, she eliminated red meat and processed food from her diet and added more fresh foods like fruits and vegetables.

She read cookbooks that taught her how to make the most of the fresh ingredients in her cooking. She also planted a garden chock-full of organic produce, including tomatoes, squash, broccoli, asparagus, and eggplant.

"I lost 12 pounds every month—ka-bam, ka-bam, ka-bam," she says. "I never even hit a plateau." In just over a year, Willson managed to take off 150 pounds. And she has maintained the weight loss ever since.

Irresistible Brussels Sprouts

FIGHTS BREAST CANCER

Hate brussels sprouts? Try this recipe, and you'll be converted.

1   package (1 pound) brussels sprouts
2   tablespoons butter
2   teaspoons Dijon mustard

Cook the brussels sprouts per package directions, then drain. Using the same pan, melt the butter and mustard over low heat. Return the sprouts to the pan and toss to coat.

Makes 4 servings

Per serving: 100 calories, 6 g fat, 3 g dietary fiber

Creamed Spinach

PREVENTS CATARACTS

Once you add a little sour cream, you won't even know that you're eating spinach.

2   packages (10 ounces each) fresh spinach
2   teaspoons butter
1   tablespoon all-purpose flour
¾   cup 1% milk
¼   cup reduced-fat sour cream
¼   teaspoon nutmeg
¼   teaspoon salt
⅛   teaspoon ground black pepper

Rinse the spinach and place it (with water still clinging to the leaves) in a large pot. Cook over medium heat until the spinach is just wilted. Drain and set aside.

Melt the butter in a small saucepan over medium heat. Whisk in the flour. Cook for 1 minute, whisking constantly.

Whisk in the milk and bring to a boil. Reduce the heat to low. Cook, whisking constantly, for 4 to 5 minutes, or until the sauce thickens. Remove from the heat.

Stir in the sour cream, nutmeg, salt, and pepper. Toss with the spinach.

Makes 4 servings

Per serving: 95 calories, 5 g fat, 4 g dietary fiber

Lima Beans They'll Love

WARDS OFF STROKE

It turns out that the perfect accompaniment for lima beans is Cheez Whiz. Who would have thought?

- 1   package (1 pound) frozen lima beans
- ¼   cup soft cheese spread (such as Cheez Whiz)
- 1   tablespoon 1% milk

Cook the lima beans per package directions. In a microwaveable bowl, melt the cheese spread and milk on high for 30 seconds. Pour it over the beans and toss.

Makes 4 servings

Per serving: 165 calories, 4 g fat, 6 g dietary fiber

Yummy Beets

THWARTS HEART ATTACKS

Most people don't like beets, but that's because of the way they are usually served. Try this recipe, and you'll be craving them once a week.

- 1   jar (16 ounces) sliced marinated beets, drained and rinsed
- ¼   cup sour cream
- 1   tablespoon chopped fresh mint
- 1   teaspoon finely chopped red onion

Place the beets in a serving bowl. Top with the sour cream, mint, and onion.

Makes 4 servings

Per serving: 87 calories, 3 g fat, 2 g dietary fiber

Really Great Veggie Sauces

Next time you're serving steamed veggies, try topping each portion with 2 tablespoons of any one of these: Hellmann's Tangerine Balsamic Citrus Splash Dressing, Ken's Steak House Lite Chunky Blue Cheese Dressing, Wish-Bone Oriental Dressing, or Hidden Valley Original Ranch Light with Sour Cream Dressing. All have 7 grams of fat or less per serving.

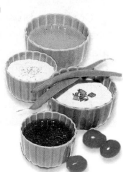

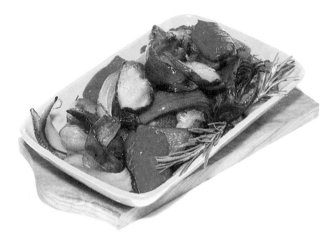

Roasted Vegetables with Olive Oil
BOOSTS IMMUNITY

Olive oil can turn any vegetable into a treat.

2	quartered red bell peppers
2	medium onions
2	zucchini cut into 2" chunks
1	tablespoon olive oil
1	teaspoon chopped fresh rosemary
1	teaspoon chopped fresh garlic
1	teaspoon balsamic vinegar
	Salt and pepper

Preheat the oven to 400°F.

Toss the bell peppers, onions, and zucchini with the olive oil. Place on a broiler pan. Roast for 30 minutes.

Toss with the rosemary, garlic, and balsamic vinegar. Add salt and pepper to taste.

Makes 4 servings

Per serving: 85 calories, 4 g fat, 4 g dietary fiber

Our Favorite Veggie Classic
FENDS OFF HEART DISEASE

The staff of *Prevention* magazine voted green bean casserole as the old-fashioned veggie classic they missed the most. Here's the slightly slimmed traditional recipe.

1	package (16 ounces) frozen french-style green beans
1	can (10¾ ounces) condensed cream of mushroom soup
¾	cup fat-free milk
⅛	teaspoon ground black pepper
1	can (3 ounces) french-fried onions

In a shallow baking dish, mix the green beans with the soup, milk, and pepper.

Bake for 30 minutes at 350°F until hot.

Sprinkle the french-fried onions on top, and bake for 5 minutes, or until the onions are golden.

Makes 5 servings

Per serving: 184 calories, 11 g fat, 4 g dietary fiber

Osteoporosis Alert

Osteoporosis isn't just for postmenopausal women. Find out why *everyone* should be concerned about this disease.

Despite the belief that osteoporosis affects only older women, an estimated 2 million American men have it, and another 3 million are at risk. Young women are also developing this bone-breaking disease in increasing numbers.

"Osteoporosis is a bigger problem than anyone believed," says John Bilezikian, M.D., director of the metabolic bone diseases program at Columbia–Presbyterian Medical Center in New York City.

One of the biggest risk factors for men is use of corticosteroid medications such as prednisone and cortisone to treat illnesses such as asthma and rheumatoid arthritis. Steroids such as these are bone robbers. For young women, chronic dieting is often the cause.

"If you find osteoporosis early and treat it, you can preserve your active, independent lifestyle," says Dr. Bilezikian. Finding the disease early means getting a bone-density test. This safe, painless, and quick test is the only way to detect bone loss before it reaches the severe stage. Don't depend on standard x-rays to do that—they pick up only a drastic bone loss of 30 percent or more.

Four Surprising Nutrients Bones Need

Old or young, male or female, osteoporosis is a concern. To prevent it, you probably know that calcium helps strengthen your bones. But did you know that at least four other vitamins and minerals might also play important supporting roles?

For example, vitamin D is essential for preventing fractures—as important, in fact, as calcium.

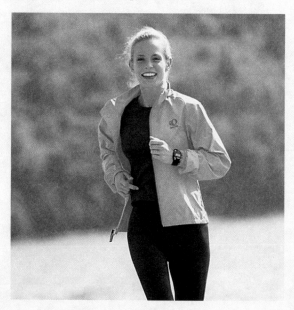

Preliminary studies also suggest that getting enough vitamin K, magnesium, and potassium could be an important bonus, says vitamin K expert Sarah Booth, Ph.D., of Tufts University in Boston.

What's troubling is that recent studies show that most people *aren't* getting enough of every single one of these nutrients. But for most of them, you can easily meet the recommended daily intake just by eating the right foods.

Let's take a closer look at what each of these nutrients does for your bones—and where you can get the amount you need.

Vitamin D. This nutrient helps your bones absorb calcium. The Daily Value is

---

QUICK & HEALTHY
HOMESTYLE HAM AND POTATO GRATIN

To make this traditionally high-fat item more nutritious while keeping its bone-building basics, fat-free milk plus just the right amount of a Swiss cheese are used. For more calcium, we've created a topping with bread crumbs and Parmesan cheese. The payoff: 349 milligrams of calcium—more than in 8 ounces of milk.

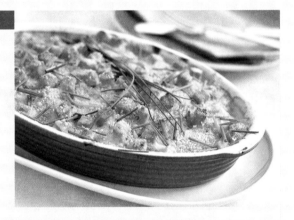

1	quart fat-free milk
2	pounds Idaho potatoes, with skin, thinly sliced
2	large cloves garlic, minced
⅔	teaspoon salt
¼	teaspoon ground red pepper
¼	cup cornstarch
12	ounces low-sodium baked ham, diced
4	ounces Gruyére or other Swiss cheese, shredded
⅓	cup chopped fresh chives or scallions
3	tablespoons unseasoned, dried whole wheat bread crumbs
3	tablespoons grated Parmesan cheese

Preheat the oven to 400°F. Combine 3⅔ cups of the milk, the potatoes, garlic, salt, and pepper in a large saucepan. Bring to a simmer. Simmer for 15 minutes, or until the potatoes are nearly tender.

While simmering, dilute the cornstarch in the remaining ⅓ cup milk. Toward the end of the simmering, stir into the potato mixture to thicken. Remove the potato mixture from the heat. Stir in the ham, Gruyére, and chives or scallions. Pour evenly into a 3-quart baking pan.

Combine the bread crumbs and Parmesan. Sprinkle over the potatoes. Bake for 15 minutes, or until the top is brown. Remove the gratin from the oven and let it sit for 12 to 15 minutes to allow it to firm up, then scoop it into portions.

Garnish with additional fresh chives, if desired. Serve with a large side salad or sautéed greens.

MAKES 8 SERVINGS
Per serving: 273 calories, 21 g protein, 30 g carbohydrates, 8 g fat, 32 mg cholesterol, 6 g dietary fiber, 710 mg sodium, 349 mg calcium

400 IU, but some experts recommend that people over age 70 get up to 600 IU. The best food sources of vitamin D are milk and some breakfast cereals. For extra insurance, consider getting more D from a multivitamin/mineral formula.

Vitamin K. This nutrient supports bone health by switching on a bone-building protein called osteocalcin. The best food sources include spinach, collard greens, coleslaw, brussels sprouts, broccoli, asparagus, and cabbage. Aim for the Daily Value of 80 micrograms.

Magnesium. A component of bone, magnesium also helps regulate blood calcium levels. The Daily Value is 400 milligrams, which you can meet by eating foods such as nuts, dried beans, crabmeat, spinach, wheat germ, wheat bran, and chocolate.

Potassium. An electrolyte, potassium may buffer acid in the blood, so it doesn't leach calcium from your bones. The Daily Value for potassium is 3,500 milligrams a day. Get yours from the most abundant sources: fruits and vegetables, salmon, lobster, milk, and yogurt.

QUICK & HEALTHY
CREAMY CAPRESE PASTA

This Italian-style pasta dish from Capri tastes like pesto, but it's creamier. Calcium-rich yogurt is the secret—and one of the reasons that this recipe is healthy for your bones.

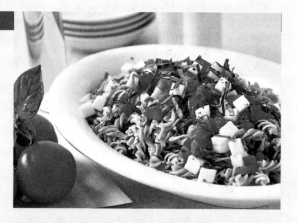

1	pound dry whole wheat pasta shapes, such as twists
1	container (8 ounces) fat-free plain yogurt
1	tablespoon + 1 teaspoon extra-virgin olive oil
½	teaspoon salt
1	large clove garlic
1	cup packed fresh basil leaves
2	large ripe tomatoes, chopped
1	teaspoon balsamic or red wine vinegar
6	ounces part-skim mozzarella cheese, cubed
	Fresh basil leaves

Prepare pasta per package directions, eliminating any suggested salt or oil.

While the pasta is boiling, place the yogurt, oil, salt, and garlic in a blender. Puree until smooth. Add the basil and puree until completely blended.

Place the tomatoes in a small mixing bowl. Toss with the vinegar and add the cheese.

Drain the pasta and place it in a large mixing bowl. Immediately pour the basil sauce over the hot pasta. Toss until the pasta is coated. Serve topped with the tomato and mozzarella mixture. Garnish with fresh basil.

MAKES 5 SERVINGS

Per serving: 475 calories, 25 g protein, 76 g carbohydrates, 11 g fat, 20 mg cholesterol, 11 g dietary fiber, 418 mg sodium

CITRUS CHICKEN BREAST with MINT and TOASTED ALMONDS

Here's a tasty twist to one of America's favorite foods—chicken. We've used calcium-fortified orange juice as a bone-building, nondairy option to create a vivid citrus sauce. As a finishing touch, we paired mint with almonds to balance the sweetness of this entrée.

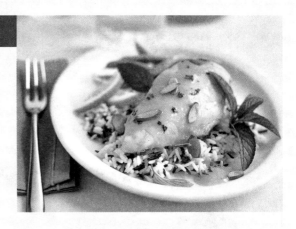

3	cups calcium-fortified orange juice
4	boneless, skinless chicken breast halves
1	medium onion, quartered
3	cloves garlic, halved
½	teaspoon salt
2	teaspoons rice wine or apple cider vinegar
2	teaspoons butter or trans-free margarine
¼	cup sliced almonds, toasted
¼	cup chopped fresh mint or 1 teaspoon dried

Place the orange juice, chicken, onion, garlic, salt, vinegar, and butter in a 2½-quart saucepan. Bring to a boil. Reduce the heat to low. Simmer for 15 minutes, or until the chicken is cooked through and the juices run clear. While the chicken is simmering, toast the almonds. (Sliced almonds can be easily toasted in a small pan over medium-high heat, stirring occasionally, for 5 minutes, or until the nuts are lightly browned.) Remove the chicken from the pan and set aside, keeping it warm.

Allow the juice to cool slightly, then puree it in a blender. Return it to the saucepan over high heat. (If using dried mint, mix it in the orange sauce while it's reducing.) Boil the mixture for 20 minutes, or until it is reduced by at least half, stirring as needed. (Reduce the heat to medium-high if the mixture begins to boil over.)

Divide the chicken among four plates. Top each piece with ¼ cup of the orange sauce. Garnish with the fresh mint and almonds. Serve the remaining sauce on the side for topping side dishes, such as brown rice pilaf and green beans or asparagus.

MAKES 4 SERVINGS

Per serving: 253 calories, 23 g protein, 24 g carbohydrates, 7 g fat, 54 mg cholesterol, 1 g dietary fiber, 344 mg sodium

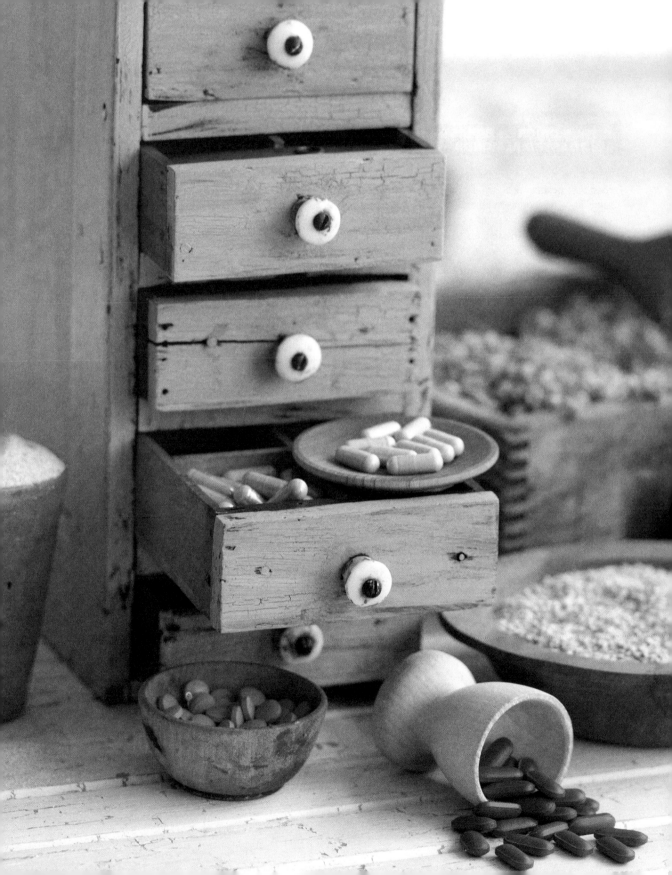

PART SEVEN

As Good As Medicine

Herbs and supplements can bolster your nutritional defense against disease.

CHAPTER 20

Your Natural Pharmacy

These 25 herbs prevent colds, double your energy, stop pain, and more.

Ever go to a health food store and feel utterly inadequate as you stare at shelf upon shelf of herbal supplements? Should you take astralagus for your fatigue or ginseng? Will echinacea cure that cold, or would goldenseal work better? Just because it costs twice as much money, is one brand of an herb twice as good as another?

Fret no more. With this simple yet comprehensive guide, you'll be armed with everything you need to know about the 25 most important supplements at the health food store. We tell you what they're used for, how much to take, and how to take it. You'll never again have to wonder why one bottle of the same herb recommends swallowing twice as many pills as another bottle. You'll be able to find all of your answers right here.

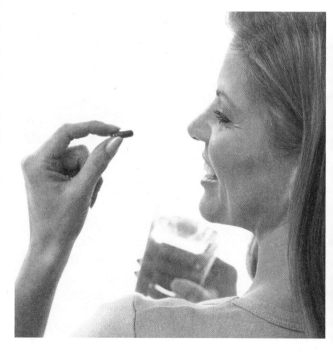

‖ Aloe

Used for: Minor burns, sunburn, minor wounds, skin ulcers, eczema, psoriasis, acne

Dosage: Apply aloe three times a day to the injured area. If you have an aloe plant, cut off a lower leaf and remove the spines. Then split the leaf in half. Apply the gel directly onto your cut, burn, wound, or breakout. Allow the gel to dry on the skin—don't wipe it off. It must remain on the skin until it dries for it to be completely effective. Your condition should improve with 2 weeks of continuous treatment.

‖ Astragalus

Used for: Immunity, colds, illness recovery, viral infections, endurance

Dosage: Astragalus must be taken continuously for 1 month before you'll see results. For this reason, herbalists often recommend using the herb for at least 3 months and for as long as 2 years. Root products have a long history of being effective, but the effectiveness of standardized extracts is less known. Take one dose three times a day.

One dose equals:

- Dried root: 1 gram in 1 cup boiled water for 10 minutes. Strain, then drink.
- 1:5 tincture: 1 teaspoon
- 1:1 tincture: 20 drops
- Dried root tablet: two 500-milligram tablets
- Standardized extract tablet: tablets containing 100 milligrams standardized to 0.5 percent 4-hydroxy-3-methoxy isoflavone

Safety with Supplements

Before you start taking any herbal or nutritional supplement, heed the following suggestions from Mark Stengler, N.D., a naturopathic doctor and author of *The Natural Physician*.

- To avoid or minimize any side effects, start with a lower dosage than the one stated on the label, then gradually increase the dosage until you reach recommended levels of the supplement.

- Consult a knowledgeable physician or health practitioner before using any new supplements. Certain herbs and nutritional supplements can be toxic when taken in higher doses.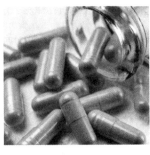

- If you are pregnant or nursing, avoid all supplements unless they have been prescribed or approved by your doctor. Also, check with your physician before using supplements if you are taking any prescription medications. People who are on anticoagulants (blood thinners), for example, should not take high doses of vitamin E, the herb red clover, or a number of other supplements that tend to thin the blood.

⌐I DID IT!

Jennifer Reid: Astralagus Helped Her Beat Chronic Fatigue

When Jennifer Reid was in her early twenties, she became sick. For almost 2 years, she could barely climb out of bed, and when she did, she'd get out of breath and become so weak that she couldn't stand up.

Different doctors tested her, first telling her that she had multiple sclerosis, then leukemia. Reid was also tested for Lyme disease and even AIDS. It was none of these. One doctor sent her to a psychologist because she was depressed.

Finally, Reid decided to take her situation in hand and do her own detective work. She started reading medical abstracts and soon realized that what she had was chronic fatigue syndrome.

She immediately made some significant changes in her diet and mental outlook. She went to an herbal shop and talked to the owner about her condition. "He suggested I try a Chinese medical formula that had astragalus as the main ingredient. He told me how astragalus has good antiviral and antibacterial components. It also helps your immune system," she said.

Reid began seeing results almost immediately, with no side effects.

"Soon I was feeling really strong," she says, "like I'd had a great boost in my immune system. Since then, I've gotten married and recently had the healthiest little baby girl. I definitely consider that visit to that herbal store to be the turning point in my recovery and my life."

‖ Black Cohosh

Used for: Irregular and painful menstruation, menopausal symptoms, fertility, mood swings

Dosage: Black cohosh needs to be used for at least three cycles—about 3 months—before you will see any results. For menopausal symptoms, take one dose three times a day. For all other conditions, take one dose twice a day.

One dose equals:

- Dried root: 1 gram in 1 cup boiled water for 10 minutes. Strain, then drink.
- 1:5 tincture: 1 teaspoon
- 1:1 tincture: 20 drops

- 4:1 dried extract tablet: one 250-milligram tablet
- Dried root tablet: two 500-milligram tablets
- Standardized extract tablet: tablets containing 1 milligram of 27-deoxyacteine

‖ Calendula

Used for: Diaper rash, athlete's foot, jock itch, nail fungus, gum health, minor cuts, burns, abrasions

Dosage: Calendula's effect is immediate, and it's safe to use long term. For internal purposes, take one dose three times a day. For external purposes, apply three or four times a day to the affected area.

One dose equals (for internal use):

- Dried flowers: 1 teaspoon in 1 cup boiled water for 10 minutes. Strain, then drink.
- 1:5 tincture: 20 drops
- 1:1 tincture: 10 drops

One dose equals (for external use):

- For gargling or topical application: 1 tablespoon of dried flowers in 1 cup boiled water for 10 minutes, then strain, or 1 teaspoon of 1:5 tincture added to 1 teaspoon water
- Cream: Mix a 4-ounce bottle of 1:5 tincture with 4 ounces of cold cream. Mix well and store in a sealed container.

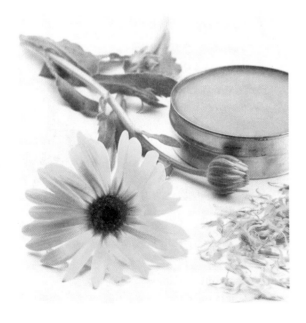

‖ Chamomile

Used for: Stomachaches, gas, irritable bowel syndrome, food poisoning, nausea, motion sickness

Dosage: The key to chamomile is to use it a lot. Take at least one dose three times a day. For chronic digestive complaints, you need to use chamomile for at least 3 months before you will see results. For temporary or occasional problems, you should feel relief within an hour.

One dose equals:

- Chamomile flowers: 1 teaspoon or 1 tea bag in 1 cup boiled water for 10 minutes. Strain, then drink.
- 1:5 tincture: 1 teaspoon
- 1:1 tincture: 20 drops

‖ Chasteberry

Used for: PMS, irregular menstruation, menopausal symptoms, low sex drive, acne, eczema, psoriasis

Dosage: For chasteberry to work effectively, you must use it for at least 3 months. It can be taken indefinitely; women often taper off after several years. Take one dose twice daily—once in the morning and once at night.

One dose equals:

- Seeds: ½ teaspoon in 1 cup boiled water for 10 minutes. Strain, then drink.
- Seed tablet: two 500-milligram tablets
- Standardized extract tablet: tablets containing 250 milligrams of 4:1 chasteberry extract
- 1:5 tincture: 60 drops
- 1:1 tincture: 12 drops

‖ Damiana

Used for: Exhaustion, mental fatigue, lack of energy, low sex drive

Dosage: Damiana increases sex drive immediately. For aphrodisiac purposes, take two doses 30 minutes before sex. Its nerve-tonic abilities kick in after about 2 weeks. For nerve-tonic purposes, take one dose three times a day.

One dose equals:
- Dried herb: 1 teaspoon in 1 cup boiled water for 3 minutes. Strain, then drink.
- 1:5 tincture: 1 teaspoon
- 1:1 tincture: 20 drops

‖ Dandelion

Used for: Toxin removal, constipation, water retention, fatigue, lack of energy

Dosage: Dandelion is very safe and can be used for extended periods of time. As a diuretic, its effects will be seen within a few hours. As a constipation remedy, it will work within 72 hours. For general health and energy, you'll need to take it for at least 1 month. For all conditions, take one dose three times a day.

One dose equals:
- Dried dandelion root: 1 teaspoon in 1 cup boiled water for 10 minutes. Strain, then drink.
- Dandelion root tablet: two 500-milligram tablets
- 1:5 tincture: 1 teaspoon
- 1:1 tincture: 20 drops

‖ Echinacea

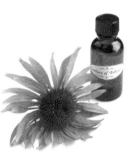

Used for: Colds and flu, infections, urinary tract infections, minor wounds

Dosage: Though safe to take long term, echinacea should be used only when needed. When you start to feel better, discontinue it. Topically, apply the tincture three times a day. Internally, take one dose three times a day.

One dose equals:
- Dried root: 1 teaspoon in 1 cup boiled water for 10 minutes. Strain, then drink.
- Dried root tablet: two 500-milligram tablets
- 1:5 tincture: 1 teaspoon
- 1:1 tincture: 20 drops

‖ Eucalyptus

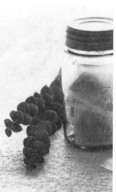

Used for: Chest and nasal congestion, colds, runny nose

Dosage: Eucalyptus can be used as long as necessary. Normally, it's discontinued once the mucus subsides. Take one dose three times a day.

One dose equals:
- Eucalyptus leaves: 1 teaspoon in 1 cup boiled water for 10 minutes. Strain, then drink.
- 1:5 tincture: 30 drops
- 1:1 tincture: 6 drops

‖ Feverfew

Used for: Migraines, chronic headaches

Dosage: Feverfew is safe to use long term, which is beneficial because people with chronic headaches and migraines need it on an ongoing basis. Do not expect to see results for at least 2 months. Take one dose every morning.

One dose equals:

- Fresh leaf: 1 leaf
- 1:5 tincture: 20 drops
- 1:1 tincture: 10 drops
- Freeze-dried leaf tablet: one 50-milligram tablet
- Standardized extract tablet: tablets containing 0.25 milligrams of parthenolide

‖ Garlic

Used for: High blood pressure, high cholesterol, heart disease, heart attack and stroke prevention

Dosage: Garlic can be used on a daily basis to undermine high blood pressure, high cholesterol, and atherosclerosis. This should be done for as long as you would like to avoid a heart attack or a stroke—in other words, forever!

In order for garlic to work, it has to be taken in large doses. The amount you get in garlic-flavored pasta sauce is not even close to a medicinal dose. To get a medicinal amount on a daily basis, use garlic supplements. If the smell of garlic bothers you, take your supplements just before bed. Otherwise, take one dose three times a day.

One dose equals:

- Fresh garlic: 4 grams (2 to 4 cloves)
- Garlic root tablet: one 500-milligram tablet

- Standardized extract tablet: tablets containing 10 milligrams of alliin or 4,000 micrograms of allicin

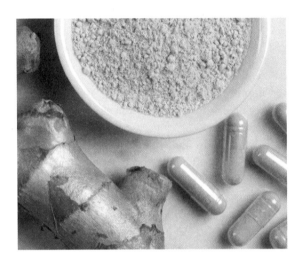

‖ Ginger

Used for: Motion sickness, nausea, food poisoning, vomiting, stomach virus

Dosage: Take one dose three times a day for as long as the digestive upset lasts. Expect relief within an hour.

One dose equals:

- Powdered dried root: ½ teaspoon in 1 cup boiled water for 10 minutes, then drink
- Fresh root: 1 teaspoon grated root in 1 cup boiled water for 10 minutes. Strain, then drink.
- 1:5 tincture: 1 teaspoon
- 1:1 tincture: 20 drops
- Ginger root tablet: two 500-milligram tablets

Ginkgo

Used for: Memory, migraines, poor circulation, impotence

Dosage: Those looking to prevent or treat poor memory, migraines, or impotence can expect to use ginkgo biloba extract on an ongoing basis. You should notice an improvement after a few weeks. To counteract the effects of the aging process, you need to use ginkgo continuously. Take one dose three times a day. Though some people report improvement after a few weeks, plan on using it for at least 4 months before developing an opinion on its effectiveness.

One dose equals:
- Standardized extract tablet: tablets containing 80 milligrams of extract standardized to 24 percent ginkgo flavone glycosides

Ginseng

Used for: Increased stamina for men, low sex drive for men, recovery from stress and illness

Dosage: As a men's tonic, ginseng must be taken for 2 months continuously before an effect will be evident. Judging its performance before that time is premature. Men should use it daily for 6 months, then 1 month off and 1 month on. As a men's tonic, take one dose each morning. For recovery from major stress or illness, take one dose daily for 6 weeks.

One dose equals:

natural WONDER

ARTICHOKE EXTRACT
Artichokes contain a compound called cynarin, which increases the liver's production of bile. That's important because bile plays a key role in the excretion of excess cholesterol from the body.

- Dried root: 1 teaspoon in 1 cup boiled water for 10 minutes. Strain, then drink.
- 1:5 tincture: 2 teaspoons
- 1:1 tincture: 40 drops
- Dried root tablet: four 500-milligram tablets
- Standardized extract tablet: tablets containing 5 milligrams of ginsenosides

Goldenseal

Used for: Urinary tract and reproductive system infections, sinusitis, tonsillitis, sore throat

Dosage: Goldenseal is recommended for infections that do not go away overnight. It must be used for at least 2 months and sometimes up to 4 months to stop the cycle of chronic infection. Take one dose three times a day.

One dose equals:
- Powdered root tablet: one 500-milligram tablet
- 1:5 tincture: 1 teaspoon
- 1:1 tincture: 20 drops

Kava

Used for: General and menopausal anxiety, nervousness, insomnia

Dosage: Kava works within 30 minutes of taking it. It can be used as a single dose, such as prior to a big meeting that is making you nervous. It can also be used on a long-term basis, such as if you are experiencing ongoing stress and anxiety. Take one dose three times a day.

One dose equals:

- Root bark: 1 gram in 1 cup boiled water for 10 minutes. Strain, then drink.
- 1:5 tincture: 1 teaspoon
- 1:1 tincture: 20 drops
- Dried root bark tablet: two 500-milligram tablets
- Standardized extract tablet: tablets containing 70 milligrams of kavalactones

Lavender

Used for: Tension, insomnia, stress and stress-related disorders

Dosage: Lavender works within a short amount of time. It is safe, so use it whenever you need it. One dose will usually do the trick, but you can have as many as three a day.

One dose equals:

- Dried lavender flowers: 1 teaspoon in 1 cup boiled water for 10 minutes. Strain, then drink.
- 1:5 tincture: 1 teaspoon
- 1:1 tincture: 20 drops
- Essential oil of lavender: 5 drops applied to the neck and shoulders. (Do not take essential oil internally.)

Maitake

Used for: Immunity, chronic infections including sinusitis, tonsillitis, bronchitis, cystitis, herpes, colds, cancer

Dosage: As with other herbal immune stimulants, maitake should be used only when necessary. If you have been diagnosed with cancer other than leukemia, take maitake for 1 month, then go off it for 1 month. Keep repeating this month-on, month-off cycle.

One dose equals:

- Fresh maitake: 1 cup cooked once a day
- Powdered, dried maitake tablet:
For prevention and immunity: six 350-milligram tablets, spread over three separate doses throughout the day
For serious illness and cancer: Eighteen 350-milligram tablets, spread over three separate doses throughout the day

Nettle

Used for: Seasonal allergies, joint inflammation, allergic skin conditions including hives and eczema

Dosage: With nettle, you won't notice a change for several weeks. Take one dose three times a day.

One dose equals:

- Dried herb: 3 grams in 1 cup boiled water for 10 minutes. Strain, then drink.
- 1:5 tincture: 1 teaspoon
- 1:1 tincture: 20 drops
- Fresh nettle juice: ½ teaspoon

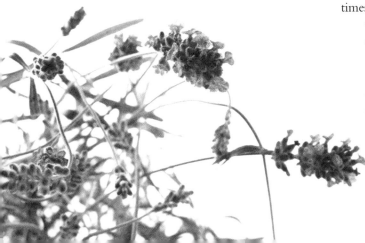

Keep or Toss?

Herbal and nutritional supplements can be an investment—and the best way to protect that investment is to store the bottles in a cool, dry place.

But what's considered a cool, dry place?

The bathroom's out because the steamy shower jacks up the humidity, and the cupboard above the stove is out because it gets hot up there. You have a lot of other choices, though.

"Keep them in a spot that's not exposed to direct sunlight, excess humidity, or heat," says V. Srini Srinivasan, Ph.D., senior scientist with the U.S. Pharmacopeia, a private standard-setting organization for the drug industry. For most people, a kitchen cupboard fits that bill, as long as it's well away from the stove.

You'll lengthen the life of your supplements if you store them in the refrigerator or freezer. If you do, though, don't leave the cap off after you take them, since moisture will condense inside the bottle. Recap the bottle quickly and return it to the refrigerator or freezer.

Some additional tips: Always keep bottles tightly closed, and don't leave supplements inside a hot car. Discard any product that begins to look or smell strange. It might have become contaminated by mold, bacteria, or other harmful organisms.

‖ Peppermint

Used for: Nausea, indigestion, weak digestion

Dosage: People from many cultures drink peppermint tea daily to keep their digestive tracts in good shape. Suffice it to say, the herb can be used long term, and to date no one has reported ill effects from doing so. To treat nausea or indigestion, take when needed. You should feel better within 30 minutes. To improve digestive function, take one dose three times a day before meals. To improve digestion in general, use for 1 month.

One dose equals:

- Fresh peppermint leaves: 1 tablespoon in 1 cup boiled water for 10 minutes. Strain, then drink.
- 1:5 tincture: ½ teaspoon
- 1:1 tincture: 10 drops

‖ St. John's Wort

Used for: Depression, burnout, nerve damage

Dosage: St. John's wort is safe for long-term treatment. Millions of people have used it year after year with no reports of ill effects. It can be taken for as long as it is needed. People often try it for a week or two, then conclude it does not work. But to feel the full effects, you must use it for at least 4 weeks and sometimes as long as 8 weeks. Don't make a judgment on its effectiveness until then. Take one dose three times a day.

One dose equals:

- Dried herb: 1 gram in 1 cup boiled water for 10 minutes. Strain, then drink.
- 1:5 tincture: 1 teaspoon
- 1:1 tincture: 20 drops
- Dried herb tablet: two 500-milligram tablets
- Standardized extract tablet: tablets containing 300 milligrams of extract standardized to 0.3 percent hypericin

‖ Saw Palmetto

Used for: Prostate problems, lack of sex drive for men, weight gain, increasing muscle mass

Dosage: Saw palmetto can and must be used for long periods of time. Take one dose three times a day.

One dose equals:
- 1:5 tincture: 1 teaspoon
- 1:1 tincture: 20 drops
- Berry tablet: two 500-milligram tablets
- Standardized extract tablet: tablets containing 100 milligrams of saw palmetto berry extract standardized to contain 85 to 95 percent fatty acids and sterols

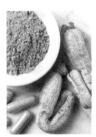

‖ Siberian Ginseng

Used for: Exhaustion, stress, lack of endurance, recovery from illness, stamina

Dosage: Siberian ginseng is nontoxic. In fact, it has been found to protect the liver from damaging toxins. Following our guidelines, you can take it for as long as you need it. Most people notice a change in their energy level after just a week. Take one dose three times a day.

One dose equals:
- Dried root bark: 1 gram in 1 cup boiled water for 10 minutes. Strain, then drink.
- 1:5 tincture: 1 teaspoon
- 1:1 tincture: 20 drops
- Dried root bark tablet: two 500-milligram tablets
- Powdered root bark tablet: two 500-milligram tablets

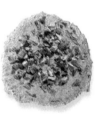

‖ Valerian

Used for: Insomnia, menstrual cramps, anxiety, tension, stress-related conditions

Dosage: Valerian can be used long term if need be. For stress and nervousness, take one dose in the morning and another in the evening. For sleep, take one dose 30 minutes before bed.

One dose equals:
- Dried valerian root: 1 gram in 1 cup boiled water for 10 minutes. Strain, then drink.
- 1:5 tincture: 1 teaspoon
- 1:1 tincture: 20 drops
- Valerian root tablet: two 500-milligram tablets
- Standardized extract tablet: tablets containing 200 milligrams of extract standardized to 0.8 percent valerianic acid

CHAPTER 21

Supplement Savvy

Here's what you need to know before you buy.

If you've read chapter 20 (Your Natural Pharmacy), you have a good idea of which herbal supplements you may want to buy. But how do you know what brand to get, and what type? Should you eat the plant? Drink it as a tea? Extract its active ingredients? Or take it as a pill or capsule?

You might have similar questions if you're shopping for nutritional supplements. What should you look for in a multivitamin? And how can you ensure that the potency lasts once you get it home? How do you know that your supplement truly contains what the bottle claims?

These are all important considerations. For answers, we turned to the experts, who gave us information that anyone taking herbs or supplements ought to know.

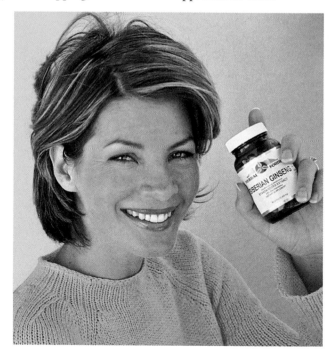

Do Dinosaurs Have What You Need?

If you have youngsters, it's possible that you have some vitamins around that are grape-flavored and resemble prehistoric cartoon characters.

Dinosaur-shaped vitamins are fine for the kids, but will they do you any good?

It's perfectly okay to take one or two each day, says Cathy Kapica, R.D., Ph.D., assistant professor of nutrition and clinical dietetics at Finch University of Health Sciences/The Chicago Medical School. In fact, if you have trouble swallowing, chewable vitamins are a reasonable way to supplement, she says. Liquid vitamins are also available, she notes.

You'll want to read labels to compare what you get in a children's vitamin to what you'd get in an adult multivitamin. This will vary by brand. If you're looking for high amounts of antioxidant nutrients, for instance, you won't find them in dinosaur-shaped, multicolored chewables. Even if you have a dinosaur as a supplement appetizer now and then, you're better off with adult-size supplements for adult-size doses, Dr. Kapica advises. Some brands even have chewables for grown-ups.

Choosing the Best Herbs

In years past, people simply added medicinal herbs to their foods, or they made some kind of brew using the dried and ground-up plant. Today, the large and small companies that distribute herbs have developed numerous ways to process them for consumption.

Three kinds of herb supplements are most common, for good reason.

Pills. The ground herb is pressed together and held by a binding substance. Some pills may have an enteric coating, a kind of second skin that's gradually dissolved by enzymes in the intestines. The coating ensures that the pill passes undisturbed through the stomach and starts to dissolve only when it reaches the intestines. Pills offer convenience, uniform doses, and specific concentrations of certain ingredients. They're also tasteless, which is sometimes

a real plus, especially if you're taking an herb like valerian. When made into a tea, valerian smells and tastes downright obnoxious. Those familiar with its rank odor have dubbed it the gym-sock herb.

Capsules. These work in much the same way as pills, but they're constructed somewhat differently. The ground herb is inside a gelatin shell, where the ingredients are protected from light, moisture, and exposure to oxygen.

Extracts. These are concentrated preparations made from dried or fresh plant parts. The herb is soaked or cooked in a liquid to concentrate active ingredients or remove unwanted components. If the active ingredient is known or suspected, manufacturers may try to include or concentrate that ingredient in their products. The content of desired constituents is calculated and standardized.

A tincture is a type of liquid extract in which alcohol is used as a solvent to extract active constituents from dried or fresh plant material. If you have difficulty swallowing pills or capsules, tinctures are a good way to go. You can simply use an eyedropper to put drops of an alcohol-based solution on your tongue, in a cup of tea, or in water.

Glycerites are a type of liquid extract in which active constituents are held in glycerin, a sweet-tasting fatty compound with a syrupy consistency. Glycerin makes herbs taste better, which can help if the raw herb is bitter or has a disagreeable flavor.

Here are some tips for choosing the best herbal pills, capsules, and extracts.

Buy the standardized extract. If you can find the supplement you want in the form of a standardized extract, it's your best assurance that the product contains a measured amount of a particular compound that's thought to be the active ingredient in the herb.

"A standardized extract gives you some guarantee that what's supposed to be in the product is probably in there. It's a good quality marker," says Alison Lee, M.D., a pain-management specialist and medical director of Barefoot Doctors, an alternative medicine practice in Ann Arbor, Michigan.

Check the botanical name. Look for the genus and species names on the product label to make sure you're getting the right herb. That's important because a common name can sometimes refer to two or three different herbs. Ginseng, for instance, is a common name, but each of three bottles of ginseng might contain a different species of the herb, and each species has different properties.

Stick with single herbs. Beware of herbal combinations and formulas, says Andrew Weil, M.D., clinical professor of internal medicine

Sizing Up Supplement Additives

In addition to the vitamins and minerals in your daily multi, you may be getting a dose of sugar, dyes, and other fillers.

These additives are also used in many drugs and aren't of concern unless you have certain food sensitivities, says V. Srini Srinivasan, Ph.D., director of dietary supplements for the United States Pharmacopeia in Rockville, Maryland, a nonprofit organization that develops and establishes standards for drugs and dietary supplements. Sugar, for instance, is required to mask the bitter taste of the ingredients. Talc or talcum powder is often added so that the pills don't stick to the machines that shape them. Starch ensures that the tablet disintegrates and dissolves once it's swallowed.

Other additives include lactose and food dyes. If you have food allergies, read the labels carefully.

and director of the program in integrative medicine at the University of Arizona College of Medicine in Tucson and author of *8 Weeks to Optimum Health*.

Herbal medication formulas take a shotgun approach, says Dr. Weil. They may expose you to more medication than you need, which makes side effects more likely.

Check expiration dates. Herbal products age rapidly with light and heat. Buy the freshest supplements you can find, says Steven Dentali, Ph.D., a natural products chemist at Dentali Associates in Troutdale, Oregon, and a member of the advisory board of the American Botanical Council.

Buy from the big guys. Large companies like Nature's Way, the Eclectic Institute, and Enzymatic Therapy have established reputations for quality control, says Dr. Weil. Without federal regulation of herbal products, you have to rely on the manufacturer for quality control.

Picking the Best Multivitamin

Beyond shaking the bottles, checking the prices, and comparing labels, how should you look for a multi?

No matter what the state of your health, it's smart to take a supplement that contains 100 percent of the Daily Value (DV) for most essential vi-

Watching the Clock

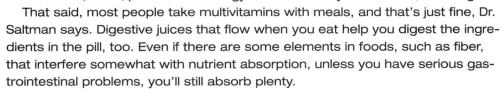

Is there a best—or worst—time to take a supplement? Yes.

When it comes to taking a multivitamin, your best bet is to keep it simple. "Just take the darn thing every day, and don't worry about where or when or with what," says Paul Saltman, Ph.D., professor of biology at the University of California, San Diego.

That said, most people take multivitamins with meals, and that's just fine, Dr. Saltman says. Digestive juices that flow when you eat help you digest the ingredients in the pill, too. Even if there are some elements in foods, such as fiber, that interfere somewhat with nutrient absorption, unless you have serious gastrointestinal problems, you'll still absorb plenty.

Here are some additional ways to optimize vitamin and mineral absorption.

- Take fat-soluble vitamins—E, D, A, and K—with a meal that contains a teaspoon or so of fat to aid absorption, says Dr. Saltman.
- Take these fat-soluble vitamins in small doses throughout the day rather than in one large dose. If you take a large, one-a-day dose, more of the vitamin is likely to be stored rather than utilized, he says.
- If you are taking a therapeutic amount of a water-soluble vitamin such as vitamin C, it's also best to divide the dose into three or more smaller doses, according to Dr. Saltman. This way, you absorb more of the vitamin, plus your blood levels of the vitamin will stay more steady throughout the day than if you take one large dose.
- Avoid taking minerals with meals that are mostly fiber, such as a high-fiber breakfast cereal, he says. As good as it is for you, fiber impairs mineral absorption.
- Minerals are also better-absorbed in divided doses, says Richard Wood, Ph.D., associate professor at Tufts University School of Nutrition in Boston. If you're taking 750 milligrams a day of calcium, for instance, you might want to try splitting it into three 250-milligram doses for midmorning, midafternoon, and before bed.

tamins and minerals. The trouble is, none of the multis contains 100 percent of what you need.

If you eat a healthful diet, you'll get many of the vitamins and minerals that you'll find in a multi, but many diets come up short on the following nutrients, experts say. You can get them by taking a multi along with a few individual supplements. Here are the suggested amounts.

- Chromium: 120 to 200 micrograms
- Copper: 2 milligrams
- Folic acid: 400 micrograms
- Magnesium: 100 milligrams
- Selenium: At least 10 micrograms
- Vitamin A/beta-carotene: 5,000 IU
- Vitamin B_6: 2 milligrams
- Vitamin D: 400 IU
- Zinc: 15 milligrams

As for iron, unless you have iron-deficiency anemia, look for a supplement that doesn't include it. You probably don't need extra iron, and studies have linked high iron levels with increased risk of heart attack and atherosclerosis (hardening of the arteries). Some premenopausal women, however, may need extra iron to compensate for menstrual blood loss.

You won't find the optimal dose of the following nutrients in any multi, so buy these supplements separately.

- Calcium: 500 to 1,000 milligrams, taken once a day.
- Vitamin C: 250-milligram tablets. The optimal dose is 500 milligrams a day, but you'll absorb more if you take two doses spaced 12 hours apart.
- Vitamin E: 100 to 400 IU, taken once a day.

CHAPTER 22

Good Pills, Bad Pills

Play it safe with these six popular over-the-counter supplements.

In Europe, where phytomedicines are common, people are accustomed to having herbs prescribed by doctors. In the United States, however, you can just walk into a health food store and buy them in quantity.

Freedom to buy what we want is part of the American way. But it doesn't come without consequences. Research shows that not all supplements actually contain the in-gredients they claim. Also, some particular types of supplements can be downright dangerous to your health, especially if you mix them with common prescription drugs.

Research has revealed a handful of supplements to be particularly problematic for a variety of reasons. Some are simply poorly understood, causing people to take the wrong supplement

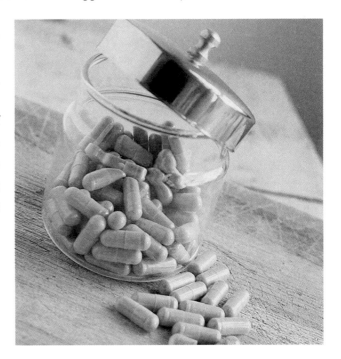

for the wrong reasons. Others contain questionable impurities. Still others are simply dangerous, especially if you have particular health concerns or take prescription drugs.

To help ensure that you stay safe, buy what you need, and get the most for your money, follow our advice for the following six problematic supplements.

‖ Ginseng

Ginseng is perhaps the most commonly used, yet most commonly misunderstood and misdirected herb on supplement store shelves. That's because there are two different types of ginseng, each with its own unique benefits. Buy the wrong type, and you'll be disappointed with the results.

Depending on its origin, *Panax ginseng* is variously known as Asian (formerly Oriental), Korean, or Chinese ginseng. American ginseng, *P. quinquefolius*, formerly grew abundantly in the wild and is now extensively cultivated in the United States and Canada. It is also grown in China. Both types of ginseng are used for their adaptogenic (tonic) effects; in other words, they gently improve general health and well-being.

The main active principles of both species of ginseng are a series of terpenoid saponins known as ginsenosides. Instead of referring to these by tongue-busting chemical names, each is designated by a capital R, followed by a letter or letter and subscript numeral. Some of these ginsenosides have very different activities, and they occur in significantly different quantities in different ginseng species. For example, Rb_1 is a

calming depressant. Rg_1, on the other hand, is a mild stimulant. In Asian ginseng, Rg_1 dominates, providing an effect that the Chinese refer to as *yang* or warm. Asian ginseng should not be used in cases of acute stress. American ginseng, on the other hand, has relatively more Rb_1, which provides an antistress effect that is called *yin* or cool.

Pick your ginseng according to the effect you desire. Need a pick-me-up? Use the Asian species. To protect yourself from stress, choose the American variety.

But be aware: Because of its relatively high price, ginseng is one of the most commonly adulterated herbs. All published studies of its quality to date have shown wide variations. Look for a product standardized on the basis of ginsenoside content. Teas prepared from authentic ginseng root (1 teaspoonful per cup) are also a good choice. Candy, chewing gum, sodas, and other nutraceutical products containing less than 1 to 2 grams of the root per serving are useless.

‖ Noni Juice

Noni juice—from the tropical plant *Morinda citrifolia*—is being touted as a treatment for diabetes, depression, high blood pressure, hemorrhoids, arthritis, even cancer. Promoters call it "an immune system miracle."

But though it's said to be an ancient Polynesian medicine, the simple truth is that there's no good information regarding its safety or effectiveness. And at least one case was reported of a man with kidney disease who, after drinking noni juice regularly, developed dangerously high

Is Your Calcium Tainted?

You may have heard about a study that found lead in 8 of 21 over-the-counter calcium carbonate supplements, and headlines warned of potential toxic lead doses. Since high levels of lead cause brain damage, of course you're worried.

But here's important information that the headlines left out: The maximum safe lead intake for people at highest risk, such as children, is 6 micrograms a day. The calcium products with lead contained only from 0.9 to 1.8 micrograms of lead per daily dose of 800 milligrams of calcium. That's well within safe limits. Besides which, calcium actually blocks the absorption of lead in the body.

But if your comfort level demands lead-free, some products with no detectable levels of lead are Nature's Bounty Oystercal-D Calcium Plus Vitamin D, Tums Ultra and Tums E-X, and Nature Made Calcium (600-milligram supplement). Another lead-free supplement is Citracal, a calcium citrate formula.

Patients with renal failure should definitely seek lead-free products, preferably by prescription.

blood levels of potassium. Turns out that noni juice is rich in potassium—about the same amount as orange juice or tomato juice, two foods that are typically forbidden for people with kidney disease.

Bottom line? There may be medicinal qualities in noni juice, but there could also be risks. If you're on a potassium-restricted diet, say no to noni.

‖ Calcium

Thanks to an array of calcium-fortified products, some people are actually overdosing on this important nutrient. The safe upper limit for calcium intake has been set at 2,500 milligrams a day. Experts think that going above that on a regular basis may invite kidney stone formation.

To make sure that you don't overdose:

Add. Total up the calcium you get in a day by looking up the percentage of the Daily Value for calcium of any food or supplement you have regularly. (To convert percentage of calcium to milligrams of calcium, drop the percent sign, and add a zero.)

Subtract. If you go over 2,500 milligrams on a regular basis (once in a while is fine), cut back. You probably need to eliminate a calcium-fortified food or supplement.

‖ Flax

Flaxseeds and products made from them contain natural hormonelike compounds called phytoestrogens that could interfere with hormone-replacement therapy.

The phytoestrogens in flaxseed are known as lignans; flaxseed has hundreds of times more lignans than any other food. "Lignans could have an estrogen-like effect on some tissues in the body and an antiestrogen effect on others," explains Sylvie Dodin, M.D., a flaxseed researcher and director of the Menopause Center at Laval University in Quebec City. But no studies have yet looked at this question.

Though there isn't a high risk to eating flaxseed while on hormone-replacement therapy, you can lower your risk by opting for lignan-free flaxseed oil. It's rich in the omega-3 fat alpha-linolenic acid, but it's virtually lignan-free because they are removed during processing. So-called high-lignan oils have some finely ground flaxseed added back, but they're still not as high in lignans as flaxseed itself.

‖ Glucosamine

Scientists have known for several years that when you inject animals with glucosamine sulfate, a popular supplement that relieves osteoarthritis pain, you trigger insulin resistance. This means that the body stops recognizing insulin and, as a result, sugar in the blood can build up to dangerous levels. But until recently, they didn't know if the same thing would happen to hu-

Testing Your Supplement

ConsumerLab.com is a new company that tests the most popular supplements to see if they actually contain the amount of ingredients that their packages say they do. According to ConsumerLab.com, the following products (bought in stores, online, and from multilevel marketers) contained levels of key ingredients lower—in some cases much lower—than the package claims.

- 6 out of 13 glucosamine/chondroitin combos (to alleviate osteoarthritis symptoms)
- 2 out of 2 chondroitin-only products (to alleviate osteoarthritis symptoms)
- 6 out of 13 SAM-e products (to relieve depression)
- 10 out of 27 saw palmetto products (for symptoms of benign prostate enlargement)
- 7 out of 30 ginkgo products (may help memory)
- 4 out of 26 vitamin C products

Fortunately, you can find out which products did pass the test—providing you with the exact contents listed on the package—by visiting www.consumerlab.com. Those products also earn the right (after paying a fee) to use the ConsumerLab.com seal of approval. So look for the distinctive logo—the letters "CL" in a laboratory beaker—on supplement products in the near future.

mans taking glucosamine. Now one small study of 15 patients with diabetes at the Los Angeles College of Chiropractic has found that taking glucosamine pills does aggravate blood sugar control.

According to Marian Parrott, M.D., vice president of clinical affairs for the American Diabetes Association, we need more research to confirm these preliminary findings. But since even a small worsening of insulin resistance can have harmful long-term consequences, diabetes experts are rightly concerned.

If you have diabetes, Dr. Parrott suggests that you consult your doctor before taking glucosamine and, if you decide to try it, check your blood sugar at least once a day during the first several days.

If you don't normally self-test, have your blood sugar checked a week or so after starting glucosamine or if you develop symptoms of hyperglycemia such as excess thirst, weakness, excess urination, weight loss, excess hunger, or blurred vision.

‖ Ephedra

Supplements containing ephedra may be helpful for certain health problems when taken under your doctor's supervision. But new evidence is leading some experts to advise staying away from ephedra as a weight-loss aid until more is known.

Neal Benowitz, M.D., professor of medicine at the University of California, San Francisco, is an independent researcher commissioned by the FDA to review 140 reports of

Be Safe Out There

Herbs generally are safer than prescription drugs, but you should always keep safety in mind. If you are under a doctor's care for any health condition or are taking medication, do not take any herb or alter your medication regimen without your doctor's knowledge. Also, do not give herbs to children without consulting a physician. And, if you are pregnant, do not self-treat with any natural remedy without the consent of your obstetrician or midwife. The same advice applies to nursing mothers and women who are trying to conceive.

adverse events related to the use of weight-loss supplements containing ephedra (also known as ma huang).

Of these cases, which include stroke, seizures, and even death in generally healthy people, one-third were definitely related to ephedra, and another one-third were possibly related.

"At present, ephedra's potential risks far outweigh its unproven benefits for weight loss. The onus is now on manufacturers to not just say but prove their products are safe with a large case-controlled study," says Dr. Benowitz. At minimum, Dr. Benowitz recommends that the FDA mandate accurate labeling and warnings on packages. (A previous study found that half of supplements contain at least 20 percent more ephedra alkaloids than what the package label says.)

Arthritis Alert

Prevention uncovers the natural remedies that can stop arthritis pain before it starts.

Your knees crackle when you stand up. Your thumbs ache. And you have that stiff, creaky shoulder thing. You don't even have much gray hair, so it couldn't be arthritis.

Or could it?

Osteoarthritis isn't supposed to happen to people in their thirties. But don't tell that to D. J. Hopwood of Tempe, Arizona. When she was 39, Hopwood was diagnosed with osteoarthritis of the spine, knees, hands, and ankles. Now 46, she's had surgery on her back, an ankle, and a knee, and she expects to need surgery on her other knee. It's just a matter of time, she says.

Now, as a volunteer and trainer for the Greater Southwest Chapter of the Atlanta-based Arthritis Foundation, Hopwood wants others to learn from her experience. Among her lessons is this nugget: Don't think that osteoarthritis strikes only the 65-plus crowd. In fact, baby boomers are at prime risk: More than half of the estimated 21 million Americans affected are under 65.

But there's no need to panic. Once you discover the disease early, there are plenty of groundbreaking treatments and natural remedies to stop it in its tracks.

A Joint Attack

Of the more than 100 types of arthritis, the most common is osteoarthritis, a joint disease that mostly affects cartilage. When cartilage breaks down, as it does in people with osteoarthritis,

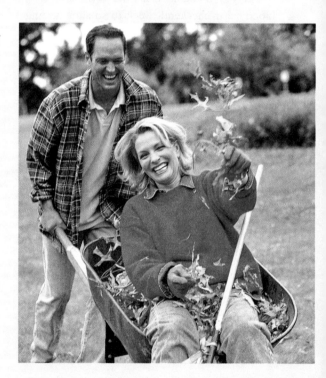

Need Help? Just Ask.

Contact the Arthritis Foundation for a free joint health kit, which includes information on preventing and controlling arthritis and a copy of the *2001 Drug Guide*. Call (800) 283-7800, or go to their Web site at www.arthritis.org. For more information on exercising away your arthritis pain (including *Prevention* magazine walking editor Maggie Spilner's tips on walking away pain), go to www.prevention.com.

bone may rub on bone, causing pain, swelling, and restricted range of motion.

In rheumatoid arthritis, which affects 2.1 million Americans, the immune system attacks the synovium, the membrane lining the joints. The resulting inflammation can damage bone and cartilage.

You can lower your risk of either type of arthritis by staying physically active, maintaining a healthy weight, and preventing injuries to your joints. Weight loss can also help if you already experience osteoarthritis, and you don't have to shed a lot of pounds to make a difference. When you walk, your knees absorb a force equal to about three times your body weight with each step. So losing just 10 pounds actually relieves each knee of about a 30-pound load with every stride you take.

Here are some other ways to ease the pain.

Eat more fish. There's strong evidence that fish—especially fish high in omega-3 fatty acids such as salmon, mackerel, brook trout, bluefish, and herring—helps decrease the risk

of rheumatoid arthritis. Eskimos and other ethnic groups who eat lots of fish are less likely to develop the condition than those who don't. One American study of 1,569 women found that those who ate two or more servings of fish a week were half as likely to develop rheumatoid arthritis as those who ate less than one serving. Researchers speculate that fish's high content of omega-3 fatty acids may affect the immune response that causes the condition.

Go vegetarian. A low-fat vegetarian diet also seems to ease arthritis symptoms. When researchers in Norway put men and women with rheumatoid arthritis on such a diet for a year, their symptoms improved significantly. Moreover, a follow-up study on this same group found that those who stayed with the plan continued to experience less pain, morning stiffness, and joint tenderness and swelling than those who returned to their regular diets.

Cut back on saturated fat. These days it's difficult to think of an illness that isn't made worse by a diet high in saturated fats. Arthritis, it appears, is no exception.

Buy Better Fish

Farm-raised salmon contain even more beneficial omega-3s than their wild cousins. It's the specially formulated feed that does it, according to the National Fisheries Institute. Plus, because they're always in season, farm-raised salmon are lower in price as well. So enjoy!

BLUE-RIBBON BLUEBERRY SOUP

This delicious soup is packed with antioxidants, thought to protect joints from the ravages of aging.

1	**quart (4 cups) fresh or frozen blueberries**
1	**cup unsweetened apple juice**
2	**tablespoons sugar**
2	**wedges lemon**
1	**stick cinnamon**
½	**teaspoon vanilla extract**
8	**tablespoons low-fat vanilla yogurt**

Place the blueberries, apple juice, sugar, lemon, cinnamon, and vanilla extract in a heavy saucepan. Bring to a boil over high heat, stirring to dissolve the sugar. Reduce the heat to low and simmer for 20 minutes.

Remove and discard the lemon wedges and the cinnamon stick.

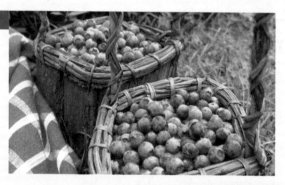

Allow the soup to cool to room temperature (about 45 minutes). Puree the soup in batches in a blender or food processor until smooth.

Chill the soup. Serve it cold, topping each serving with 2 tablespoons of the yogurt.

MAKES 4 SERVINGS

Per serving: 155 calories, 2 g protein, 37 g carbohydrates, 1 g fat, 2 mg cholesterol, 3 g dietary fiber, 31 mg sodium

In one study, 23 people with rheumatoid arthritis were put on a very low fat (10 percent of calories from fat) diet for 12 weeks. They also walked 30 minutes a day and followed a stress-reduction regimen. People in this group experienced a 20 to 40 percent reduction in joint tenderness and swelling; many of them were able to cut back on arthritis medications. People in a second group who didn't follow the diet showed no such improvement.

"We think that the diet caused most of the improvements in joint swelling and tenderness," says study leader Edwin H. Krick, M.D., associate professor of medicine at Loma Linda University in California.

A diet low in saturated fats reduces the body's production of prostaglandins, hormonelike substances that contribute to inflammation, says Dr. Krick. In addition, a low-fat diet may hinder communications sent by the immune system, thereby interrupting the body's inflammatory response. "Interrupting those chemicals can help the joints get better," he says. "One way to accomplish that is by consuming a low-fat or largely vegetarian diet."

Focus on vitamin C. Researchers at Boston University School of Medicine studied the eating habits of people with osteoarthritis of the knee. They found that those getting the most vitamin C—more than 200 milligrams a day—

were three times less likely to experience worsening of the disease than those who got the least vitamin C (less than 120 milligrams a day).

The researchers aren't sure why vitamin C seemed to make such a difference, says study leader Timothy McAlindon, M.D., assistant professor of medicine at the medical school. Since vitamin C is an antioxidant, it may protect the joints from the damaging effects of free radicals, unstable molecules that can cause joint inflammation. "Vitamin C may also help generate collagen, which enhances the body's ability to repair damage to the cartilage," he says.

natural
WONDER
EXTRA-VIRGIN OLIVE OIL
In a recent Greek study, those with the lowest lifetime consumption of extra-virgin olive oil were 2½ times more likely to develop rheumatoid arthritis than those with the highest.

Dr. McAlindon recommends that people get at least 120 milligrams of vitamin C a day in their diets, twice the Daily Value. "That's the amount in a couple of oranges," he says. Other fruits and vegetables rich in vitamin C include cantaloupe, broccoli, strawberries, peppers, and cranberry juice.

Go for immunity boosters. To boost your immune system, eat whole grains, green leafy vegetables, seafood, lean meats, and moderate amounts of vegetable oils to get vitamins B_6 and E, and the trace mineral zinc. Your body will be better able to fight infections and chronic disease with these nutrients.

I DID IT!

Take a Lesson from Broadway Joe's Knees

Quarterbacks take a beating on the field, and Joe Namath was certainly no exception. Today, the former New York Jets star suffers from osteoarthritis of the knees, spine, and thumb as a result of years of twisting, turning, stopping, and starting on the football fields he called home for most of his young life.

"Football is a great sport, but the body wasn't designed for it," says Namath, who retired in 1977. He had both knees replaced in 1992, making it easier to lift his two young daughters without fear of falling down. The surgery also took away the pain, which was "always there, always in the back of my mind," he says.

Today, Namath lifts weights and works out on an elliptical exercise machine, a combination stairclimber and cross-country skiing device that goes easy on his knees and spine.

Arthritis will get worse if you don't take care of your body, he warns. "I know that it's hard to change habits. For people who may not have worried about diet or exercise for most of their lives, it's hard to get into a healthy lifestyle. But it's not impossible. You have to make it a priority."

Guidelines for Safe Self-Care

Herbs

While herbal home remedies are generally safe and cause few, if any, side effects, herbalists are quick to caution that botanical medicines should be used cautiously and knowledgeably.

Most important, if you are under a doctor's care for any health condition or are taking any medication, do not take any herb or alter your treatment regimen without informing your doctor. Do not administer herbs to children without consulting a physician. Also, if you are pregnant, nursing, or attempting to conceive, do not self-treat with any natural remedy without the consent of your obstetrician or midwife. Some herbs may cause adverse reactions if you are allergy-prone, have a major health condition, take prescription medication, take an herb for too long, take too much, or use the herb improperly. Homeopathic remedies are generally considered safe.

The guidelines in this chart are intended for adults only and usually refer to internal use. Be aware that some herbs may cause a skin reaction when applied topically. If you are trying an herb for the first time, it is always wise to do a patch test. Put a small amount on your skin and observe the exposed area for 24 hours to be sure that you aren't sensitive. If redness or a rash occurs, discontinue use.

Due to reports that some Chinese-made products contain potentially harmful contaminants, it is recommended that you obtain Chinese herbal remedies from a qualified practitioner of Traditional Chinese Medicine. While Ayurvedic herbs do not pose the same concern, it is best to consult an Ayurvedic practitioner to obtain the highest-quality herbs and receive personalized recommendations regarding their safe use. (Note: mg = milligrams)

206

Herb	Safe Use Guidelines and Possible Side Effects
Aloe	Do not apply the gel to any surgical incision, because it may delay healing. The dried form of the gel is a habit-forming laxative and should not be ingested. The fresh juice is generally regarded as safe for internal use.
Ashwaganda	Do not use with barbiturates; it may intensify their effects.
Black cohosh	Do not use for more than 6 months.
Cascara sagrada	Do not use if you have an inflammatory condition of the intestines, an intestinal obstruction, or abdominal pain. Do not use for more than 14 days; it may cause laxative dependency and diarrhea.
Chamomile	Very rarely, may cause an allergic reaction when ingested. Drink the tea with caution if you are allergic to closely related plants, such as ragweed, asters, and chrysanthemums.
Chasteberry (vitex)	May counteract the effectiveness of birth control pills.
Dandelion	If you have gallbladder disease, do not use dandelion root preparations unless under the supervision of a knowledgeable medical doctor.
Echinacea	Do not use if you are allergic to closely related plants, such as ragweed, asters, and chrysanthemums. Do not use if you have tuberculosis or an autoimmune condition such as lupus or multiple sclerosis, because echinacea stimulates the immune system.
Ephedra (ma huang)	Use only under the guidance of a qualified practitioner.
Feverfew	Chewing the fresh leaves can cause mouth sores in some people.
Flaxseed	May affect the absorption of drugs; take only under the supervision of a knowledgeable medical doctor if you're on any medication. Do not use the seeds if you have a bowel obstruction. Otherwise, take the seeds with at least 8 ounces of water. Flaxseed oil is generally regarded as safe.
Garlic	Do not use garlic supplements if you are taking anticoagulants (blood thinners) or if you're about to undergo surgery; the supplements thin the blood and may increase bleeding. Likewise, fresh garlic should be limited to two cloves a day if you are taking anticoagulants or if you're about to undergo surgery. Do not use garlic in any form if you are taking drugs to lower blood sugar.
Ginger	If you have gallstones, do not use therapeutic amounts of dried root or powder unless under the supervision of a knowledgeable medical doctor; it may increase bile secretion.
Ginkgo	Do not use with antidepressant MAO inhibitors such as phenelzine sulfate (Nardil) or tranylcypromine (Parnate), aspirin or other nonsteroidal anti-inflammatory drugs, or blood-thinning medications such as warfarin (Coumadin). May increase dermatitis, diarrhea, and vomiting in doses exceeding 240 mg of concentrated extract.
Ginseng (American, Asian)	Do not use if you have high blood pressure. May cause irritability if taken with caffeine or other stimulants.
Goldenseal	Do not use internally if you have high blood pressure or if you are pregnant.
Kava	Stay within the dosage recommendations on the label. Do not use with alcohol or barbiturates. Because kava is a muscle relaxant, exercise caution when driving or operating equipment.

Herb *(cont.)*	Safe Use Guidelines and Possible Side Effects *(cont.)*
Licorice	Do not use if you have diabetes, high blood pressure, a liver or kidney disorder, or a low potassium level. Do not use daily for more than 4 to 6 weeks; overuse can lead to water retention, high blood pressure caused by potassium loss, or impaired heart and kidney function.
Myrrh	May cause diarrhea and irritate the kidneys. Do not use if you have uterine bleeding.
Nettle	May cause allergy symptoms to worsen. If you have allergies, take only one dose a day for the first few days.
Rosemary	May cause excessive menstrual bleeding in therapeutic amounts. Considered safe when used as a seasoning.
Sage	May increase the sedative effects of drugs when taken in therapeutic amounts. Do not use if you are hypoglycemic or undergoing anticonvulsant therapy.
St. John's wort	Do not use with antidepressants unless under the supervision of a knowledgeable medical doctor. Avoid direct sunlight during treatment; St. John's wort may increase the skin's sensitivity to sun exposure.
Saw palmetto	Do not use to treat an enlarged prostate without first consulting your doctor.
Turmeric	Do not use in therapeutic amounts if you have high stomach acid or ulcers, gallstones, or a bile duct obstruction.
Valerian	May intensify the effects of sleep-enhancing or mood-regulating medications. May cause heart palpitations and nervousness in people who are sensitive to it. If such stimulant action occurs, discontinue use.

Vitamins and Minerals

Although reports of toxicity from vitamins and minerals are rare, they do occur. The information here is designed to help you use vitamins and minerals safely. The doses mentioned below are not recommendations; rather, they are the levels at which harmful side effects can occur. Keep in mind that significantly lower levels may cause problems in some people.

For best absorption and minimal stomach irritation, take supplements with a meal unless otherwise indicated. It's important to realize that supplements are not substitutes for a healthy diet, since they do not provide all the nutritional benefits of whole foods.

If you have a serious chronic illness that requires continual medical supervision, always talk to your doctor before self-treating. And even if you're perfectly healthy, you should always tell your doctor which supplements you're taking. That way, if you need medication for any reason, your doctor can give you a prescription without putting you at risk for a dangerous drug interaction. If you are pregnant, nursing, or attempting to conceive, do not take supplements without a doctor's supervision. (Note: mg = milligrams; mcg = micrograms; IU = international units)

Nutrient	Safe Use Guidelines and Possible Side Effects
B-complex vitamins	Do not exceed the dosage recommended on the label.
Calcium	Do not exceed 2,500 mg a day unless under the supervision of a knowledgeable medical doctor. Some natural sources of calcium, such as bonemeal and dolomite, may be contaminated with lead.
Chromium (all forms)	Do not exceed 1,000 mcg a day unless under the supervision of a knowledgeable medical doctor.
Copper	Do not exceed 10 mg a day unless under the supervision of a knowledgeable medical doctor.
Folic acid	Do not take more than 1,000 mcg a day unless under the supervision of a knowledgeable medical doctor.
Iron	For most people, doses exceeding 25 mg a day should be taken only under medical supervision. The maximum daily dose for men and postmenopausal women is 8 mg.
Magnesium (all forms)	Consult your doctor before beginning supplementation if you have heart or kidney problems. Doses exceeding 350 mg a day may cause diarrhea.
Niacin (all forms)	Do not exceed 35 mg a day unless under the supervision of a knowledgeable medical doctor.
Potassium	Take only under the supervision of a knowledgeable medical doctor.
Selenium	Do not exceed 400 mcg a day unless under the supervision of a knowledgeable medical doctor.
Vitamin A	Do not exceed 10,000 IU a day unless under the supervision of a knowledgeable medical doctor. Larger doses may cause vomiting, fatigue, dizziness, and blurred vision.
Vitamin B_6	Do not exceed 100 mg a day unless under the supervision of a knowledgeable medical doctor. Larger doses may cause nerve damage, resulting in a tingling sensation in the fingers and toes. Other possible side effects include pain, numbness, weakness in the limbs, depression, and fatigue.
Vitamin C	Doses exceeding 2,000 mg a day may cause diarrhea.
Vitamin D	Do not exceed 2,000 IU a day unless under the supervision of a knowledgeable medical doctor.
Vitamin E	Do not exceed 1,500 IU (natural form) or 1,100 IU (synthetic form) a day unless under the supervision of a knowledgeable medical doctor. Because vitamin E acts as a blood thinner, consult your doctor before beginning supplementation in any amount, if you're already taking aspirin or a blood-thinning medication such as warfarin (Coumadin).
Vitamin K	Take only under the supervision of a knowledgeable medical doctor.
Zinc	Do not exceed 40 mg a day unless under the supervision of a knowledgeable medical doctor.

Emerging Supplements

Reports of adverse effects from emerging supplements are rare, especially in comparison with prescription drugs. You should be aware, however, that many of these supplements have little scientific research to assess their safety or long-term effects. What's more, some supplements can complicate existing conditions or cause allergic reactions in some people. For these reasons, you should always check with your doctor before beginning supplementation of any kind.

Supplement manufacturers are required by law to provide information on their product labels about reasonably safe recommended dosages for healthy individuals. For these newer supplements, many experts advise you to follow the label directions.

In addition, we suggest that you take supplements with food to avoid stomach irritation. Never use them as substitutes for a healthy diet, since they do not provide all the nutritional benefits of whole foods. And, if you are pregnant, nursing, or attempting to conceive, do not take supplements without a doctor's supervision. (Note: g = grams; mg = milligrams)

Supplement	Safe Use Guidelines and Possible Side Effects
Arginine (L-arginine)	May cause nausea and diarrhea in large doses. May increase outbreaks in those who have genital herpes. Do not use with lysine; the two supplements compete for absorption in the body. Arginine's long-term effects are unknown.
Bromelain	May cause nausea, vomiting, diarrhea, skin rash, and heavy menstrual bleeding. May increase the risk of bleeding in those taking aspirin or anticoagulants (blood thinners). Do not use if you are allergic to pineapple.
Glucosamine	May cause upset stomach, heartburn, or diarrhea.
Lactobacillus acidophilus	Doses exceeding 10 billion viable organisms a day may cause mild gastrointestinal distress. Consult your doctor before beginning supplementation if you have any serious gastrointestinal problems that require medical attention. If you are using antibiotics, take them at least 2 hours before the supplements.
Omega-3 fatty acids	In some people, doses as small as 2 g a day may reduce the blood's clotting ability, resulting in bleeding or, in extreme instances, hemorrhaging.
Quercetin	In some people, doses exceeding 100 mg a day may dilate blood vessels and thin the blood. Do not use if you're at risk for low blood pressure or you have problems with blood clotting.
SAM-e	May increase blood levels of homocysteine, a significant risk factor for cardiovascular disease.

Essential Oils

Essential oils are inhaled or applied topically to the skin. With few exceptions, they are never taken internally.

Of the most common essential oils, lavender, tea tree, lemon, sandalwood, and rose can be used undiluted. The rest should be diluted in a carrier base—which can be an oil (such as almond), a cream, or a gel—before being applied to the skin.

Many essential oils may cause irritation or allergic reactions in people with sensitive skin. Before applying any new oil to your skin, always do a patch test. Put a few drops of the essential oil, mixed with the carrier, on the back of your wrist and wait for an hour or more. If irritation or redness occurs, wash the area with cold water. In the future, use half the amount of essential oil or avoid it altogether.

Do not use essential oils at home for serious medical problems. During pregnancy, do not use essential oils unless they're approved by your doctor. Essential oils are not appropriate for children of any age.

Store essential oils in dark bottles, away from light and heat and out of the reach of children and pets.

Essential Oil	Safe Use Guidelines and Possible Side Effects
Eucalyptus	Do not use for more than 2 weeks without the guidance of a qualified practitioner. Do not use more than 3 drops in bathwater. Do not use at the same time as homeopathic remedies. Do not apply to the faces of infants and young children.
Lavender	Keep the undiluted oil away from your eyes.
Peppermint	Do not use more than 3 drops in bathwater. Do not use at the same time as homeopathic remedies. Do not apply to the faces of infants and small children. Keep the oil away from your eyes. It can be taken internally, but it may cause stomach upset in sensitive individuals. Do not ingest the oil without medical supervision if you have gallbladder or liver disease.

Credits

Cover photograph
Hilmar

Interior photographs

Beth Bischoff: 52

CMCD: 195, 196

Corel: 75

Courtesy Photo: 84

Digital Vision, Ltd.: 10, 21 *(left)*, 46

G&M David de Lossy/Image Bank: 32

Brian Hagiwara: 13 *(right)*, 14 *(left)*, 39, 41, 43, 45, 49, 53, 78, 101, 141, 143, 162 *(bottom)*, 164 *(top)*, 171, 172, 174, 175

John Hamel/Rodale Images: 44, 97, 109, 122, 136

Hilmar: xiii, xiv, 2, 15, 16, 22 *(right)*, 24, 28, 30, 34, 36, 38, 50, 54, 56, 62, 64, 70, 73, 74, 80, 83, 86, 88, 91, 94, 100, 106, 108, 110, 112, 113, 114, 115, 116, 118, 121, 123, 125, 128, 130, 134, 138, 139, 140, 142, 146, 150, 152, 156, 160, 166, 168, 176, 192, 202

Walter Hodges/Stone: 60

Mitch Mandel/Rodale Images: 18 *(left)*, 85, 93, 129 *(right)*, 148, 157, 183 *(left)*, 185, 186 *(top and middle)*, 191 *(right)*

Rita Maas: 177, 178, 179

Alison Miksch: 7

Luciana Pampalone: 197

Photodisc: 6 *(right)*, 11, 17 *(top)*, 20, 21 *(right)*, 22 *(left)*, 23, 25, 26, 59, 103, 119, 183 *(right)*, 187, 191 *(left)*

Todd Powell: 133

Howard Puckett: 67

Rodale Images: 5 *(right)*, 6 *(left)*, 9, 14 *(right)*, 19, 47, 98, 170, 186 *(bottom)*, 190, 204

John Sterling Ruth: 18 *(right)*, 76, 124, 165 *(bottom)*

Margaret Skrovanek/Rodale Images: 48

Tim Sloan: 144

Christie Tito/Rodale Images: 17 *(bottom)*

Jimmy Williams: 137

Kurt Wilson/Rodale Images: 3, 5 *(left)*, 8, 12, 13 *(left)*, 29, 37, 68, 77, 95, 120, 129 *(left)*, 135, 154, 155, 161, 162 *(top)*, 163, 164 *(bottom)*, 165 *(top left and right)*, 180, 182, 189

Alan Wycheck/Liaison Agency: 104

Index

Underscored page references indicate boxed text. **Boldface** references indicate photographs.

Conversion Chart

These equivalents have been slightly rounded to make measuring easier.

VOLUME MEASUREMENTS

U.S.	Imperial	Metric
¼ tsp	–	1 ml
½ tsp	–	2 ml
1 tsp	–	5 ml
1 Tbsp	–	15 ml
2 Tbsp (1 oz)	1 fl oz	30 ml
¼ cup (2 oz)	2 fl oz	60 ml
⅓ cup (3 oz)	3 fl oz	80 ml
½ cup (4 oz)	4 fl oz	120 ml
⅔ cup (5 oz)	5 fl oz	160 ml
¾ cup (6 oz)	6 fl oz	180 ml
1 cup (8 oz)	8 fl oz	240 ml

WEIGHT MEASUREMENTS

U.S.	Metric
1 oz	30 g
2 oz	60 g
4 oz (¼ lb)	115 g
5 oz (⅓ lb)	145 g
6 oz	170 g
7 oz	200 g
8 oz (½ lb)	230 g
10 oz	285 g
12 oz (¾ lb)	340 g
14 oz	400 g
16 oz (1 lb)	455 g
2.2 lb	1 kg

LENGTH MEASUREMENTS

U.S.	Metric
¼"	0.6 cm
½"	1.25 cm
1"	2.5 cm
2"	5 cm
4"	11 cm
6"	15 cm
8"	20 cm
10"	25 cm
12" (1')	30 cm

PAN SIZES

U.S.	Metric
8" cake pan	20 × 4 cm sandwich or cake tin
9" cake pan	23 × 3.5 cm sandwich or cake tin
11" × 7" baking pan	28 × 18 cm baking tin
13" × 9" baking pan	32.5 × 23 cm baking tin
15" × 10" baking pan	38 × 25.5 cm baking tin (Swiss roll tin)
1½ qt baking dish	1.5 liter baking dish
2 qt baking dish	2 liter baking dish
2 qt rectangular baking dish	30 × 19 cm baking dish
9" pie plate	22 × 4 or 23 × 4 cm pie plate
7" or 8" springform pan	18 or 20 cm springform or loose-bottom cake tin
9" × 5" loaf pan	23 × 13 cm or 2 lb narrow loaf tin or pâté tin

TEMPERATURES

Fahrenheit	Centigrade	Gas
140°	60°	–
160°	70°	–
180°	80°	–
225°	105°	¼
250°	120°	½
275°	135°	1
300°	150°	2
325°	160°	3
350°	180°	4
375°	190°	5
400°	200°	6
425°	220°	7
450°	230°	8
475°	245°	9
500°	260°	–